THE PREMED PARADOX

What You Need to Know About the Life of a Physician

AMIT PANDEY, MD

Copyright © 2023 Amit Pandey
All rights reserved

The details of clinical encounters in this book were omitted to protect patient privacy.

No part of this book may be reproduced, or stored in a retrieval system, or transmitted in any form or by any means, electronic, mechanical, photocopying, recording, or otherwise, without express written permission of the author.

Print book ISBN: 979-8-218-30492-8
Book design by: Andy Magee
www.thepremedparadox.com

To my incredible peers in the healthcare field and the determined generations of aspiring premeds that will follow us. Your tireless work and noble motivations are what keep our patients—and our healthcare system—alive.

Acknowledgements

There are many individuals I must take the time to thank, as they were instrumental in helping me achieve my goal of writing this book.

First, I must thank my wife, Ruchi Vig. Without her love and support each day, as well as her excellent input throughout the process, I never could have completed this project. She has supported me through most of my medical journey, which certainly has not been easy, and for that I will forever be grateful.

Next, I would like to thank my family, specifically my parents, Dr. Braj Pandey and Manjula Pandey. Their love and guidance have helped me become who I am today, and their feedback at the final stages of completing my book was crucial.

I would also like to acknowledge the several mentors throughout my career who have guided me and set the example of what a good professional, clinician, and person looks like.

I must also thank my countless colleagues and peers in the medical field with whom I have discussed many topics that were essential to this book. They have inspired me to put pen to paper and complete this text in order to pay it forward to future generations of aspiring physicians.

Many thanks my editor, Rebecca Raskin, and my book designer, Andy Magee. Without their expertise and skill, this book could never have reached the level of quality that it did in the end.

And finally, I would like to thank an intelligent and ambitious group of aspiring physicians who provided feedback on this book: Pranay Narang, Nikhil Sinha, and Arushi Rai. Their ideas and perspectives helped me refine this project and make it most useful for those who need it most.

My sincere thanks to you all. I could not have done this without you.

Table of Contents

Part I: Prelude

Chapter 1:	Paradox	3
Chapter 2:	Ignorance and Inertia	11
Chapter 3:	Duality	15

Part II: Preparation

Chapter 4:	Why Medicine?	30
Chapter 5:	Is Medicine Right for Me?	45
Chapter 6:	Types of Physician Degrees	62
Chapter 7:	Alternative Career Paths Within Healthcare	72

Part III: Pursuit

Chapter 8:	What is Premed Really Like?	88
Chapter 9:	What is Medical School Really Like?	98
Chapter 10:	What is Residency Really Like?	120

Part IV: Practice

Chapter 11:	What is Attending Life Really Like?	148
Chapter 12:	Financial Implications of a Career as a Physician	164
Chapter 13:	Common Challenges of a Career as a Physician	178
Chapter 14:	Psychological and Emotional Impacts of a Career as a Physician	186
Chapter 15:	Burnout	203

Part V: Postscript

Chapter 16: A Reflection on COVID-19 – What We Have Learned from the Global Pandemic	214
Chapter 17: A Tale of Two Premeds	229
References	239
About the Author	248

Part I: Prelude

Chapter 1: Paradox

See one. Do one. Teach one. This timeless saying is a central slogan in the world of medicine, a badge of honor carried proudly on the road to becoming a physician. It refers to the process of learning to do something new, which we do often as physicians: observing someone else completing a task (see one); performing the task yourself under supervision (do one); and quickly becoming an expert, such that you can educate others on how to do the same (teach one).

This is an oversimplification, of course, particularly in the case of learning new procedures or technical skills to be performed on the human body. The reality is that modern medical and surgical education now rely much more on evidence, supervised repetition, and even technological simulation. Some surgical residencies require six or more years of intense training to develop the expertise needed to cut human flesh and heal patients. But the see one, do one, teach one approach is still essential to the life of a physician: medicine encourages you to dive into the deep end, to take action, to get your hands dirty (quite literally), and to learn by doing.

I vividly remember experiencing this progression on my road to becoming a physician. "Doing one" for the first time, getting to truly treat patients and perform procedures, was both nerve-wracking and exhilarating. Sometimes our most memorable moments are the most humbling ones. These experiences help us develop a healthy respect for the challenges that come with caring for human lives. One such memory is the first time I performed a procedure called a paracentesis.

I had recently graduated from medical school and been granted the title "intern," which (in the medical world) means a first-year resident. Most of my days were spent nervously but excitedly scurrying around the hospital, examining patients, ordering medications, performing procedures, and learning a ton along the way. Each day brought unique cases and brand-new experiences. The pace was fast and relentless, which made it both exciting and stressful at the same time.

One afternoon, after we had finished seeing our patients as a team, my patient needed a paracentesis—a procedure in which a needle is used to extract fluid from the abdomen. He had liver scarring called cirrhosis, which often leads to the accumulation of abdominal fluid, which in turn can cause pain, shortness of breath, or infection. I had learned the theory and technique of this procedure through a teaching session, which concluded with practicing on a simulated model. I had also observed my senior residents performing the procedure before. Now that I had completed the "see one" step, it was time to step up to the plate and "do one."

My logical mind felt prepared. But, as I grabbed the necessary equipment and began making my way to the patient's floor, a thick cloud of anxiety hovered over me. Performing procedures on real, live patients was different than simulated teaching sessions. The stakes, and consequences, were much higher.

I have always respected the responsibility of placing a needle or scalpel on the human body. Along with this respect, I still had the nerves that came with limited experience and just a bit of self-doubt. I clenched my clammy palms and felt a flutter in my chest as I strolled through the hallway toward the patient's room.

But we are all beginners at some point, I thought to myself. *No one is born an expert. I have to be bold. I have to embrace these moments to learn and grow.*

My supervising physician, the head of the team, had accompanied me to the patient's bedside to oversee and support me through the procedure.

"You've done one of these before, right?" I remember him asking in a somewhat nonchalant manner, perhaps expecting a casual "yes" in response.

"No," I replied, a bit sheepishly. "Not on a real patient. But I've learned in training and practiced on a model. I should be good to go." I was unsure if the confidence I was trying to portray was coming across. The truth was that I *did* know what I was doing. I had studied the technique quite closely. But confidence is often borne out of experience. I was well on my way, but I needed practice to build comfort and proficiency.

"Alright," he sighed, the slightest hint of exasperation in his tone. "I'll be here if you need me." He had probably just realized that more would be required of him than simple observation. I was a newly minted intern after all. It might be time for him to teach.

As we entered the room, I greeted the patient and explained to him what we would be doing during the procedure. He quickly nodded in agreement. He was excited to rid himself of the fluid which was causing abdominal pain and shortness of breath. I began to arrange my workspace, setting down the paracentesis kit and all the materials needed to perform the procedure: needle, scalpel, catheter, sterilization tools, and bottles to collect the fluid. I took a moment to remind myself of the steps of the procedure, which I had memorized several times over. With a deep breath to steady my nerves, I peeled back the adhesive seal of the kit and got to work.

After positioning the patient, using an ultrasound to identify the safest location to place the needle, and sterilizing the field, I was ready for action. The next step seemed quite innocuous to me; but in retrospect, I should not have overlooked it. It was time to inject the patient with a numbing medication called lidocaine, via a small needle, to desensitize the area and prevent pain when the larger needle and catheter were placed into the abdominal wall. This procedure kit came with a glass lidocaine vial with a tip that needed to be broken to open it and access the medication inside. When doing so, one typically uses a sterile towel or sterile gauze to crack the tip of the vial and prevent injury or cuts to one's own skin.

As I had seen my senior residents do in the past, without a second thought, I picked up the sterile gauze, folded it over to create a padded protection from the glass of the vial, and snapped off the top as required. To my absolute shock, I immediately felt the glass tip of the vial penetrate both gauze padding and sterile glove, cleanly slicing through my thumb which had applied the pressure. I placed the lidocaine bottle back on the kit and looked down, horrified, as round drops of bright red blood began to emerge from the slit in my pearly white glove. I looked over to the supervising doctor who was standing behind me, and barely managed to croak out these five words: "I think I cut myself."

I was about ten minutes into my first ever procedure as an internal medicine intern, and I had injured myself before even touching the patient. I had no choice: I was forced to abort the procedure, clean up, and first stop the bleeding in my finger before I could proceed with anything else. I apologized to the patient, attempting to hide my emotions. I don't think I had ever been more professionally embarrassed.

Luckily, the patient and my supervising doctor were quite gracious. "Mistakes happen," they said. The patient was doing just fine. "No problem, and no harm done." Their support and patience meant more than they knew.

Once I had cleaned and stabilized the cut, I gathered my courage and returned to the patient. I was able to start once again and successfully complete the procedure. The irony (and relief) is that everything with the patient went perfectly. The second time around, though my anxiety was heightened by my previous failure, my hands were steady. The needle passed easily into the patient's belly, clear-yellow fluid flowing out without resistance. The patient had no discomfort, and things went as smoothly as I could have hoped for. He felt much better afterwards and thanked me for my efforts, with a bit of a knowing smile that comes with witnessing such a memorable misstep.

I have since done that procedure and others countless times during my time as an internal medicine physician, but I have never had such a humbling experience. In that moment, with that simple mistake, I had a shocking realization which proved to be an invaluable lesson: the practice of medicine is difficult and unpredictable, and I was in for the ride of a lifetime. No matter how prepared I thought I was, I would face unexpected challenges and failures along the way. That would be a part of the process, and the hard times would probably teach me more than any other. In order to traverse the medical education gauntlet, I would be put in countless new and uncomfortable situations. But humility—understanding that there is so much to learn and no one can ever be fully prepared—would be perhaps the biggest lesson I would learn as a medical trainee.

Looking back, in this moment of perceived failure, I was able to rely on my education and training to ultimately succeed. Having seen and learned the procedure before allowed me to regroup, bounce back from my initial misstep, and eventually execute successfully to treat the patient. This is why the "see one, do one, teach one" concept survives to this day. Education and exposure lead to experience which in turn leads to expertise. The slogan lives on in the heart and soul of the medical community because it captures our essence: embracing the challenge and bravely pushing on during tough times to master the crucial skills of healing.

If we take a step back and apply this slogan to medical training as a whole, to the process of *becoming a physician*, the concept again holds truth. Premeds also have a tendency to jump right in, to commit themselves fully, to dive head-first into their future endeavors on the way to becoming a doctor.

The medical education process is rigorous. It demands this wholehearted and unwavering commitment. I commend the bravery and dedication of anyone who chooses to pursue a career as a physician. It is an amazing but challenging pursuit, filled with experiences spanning the emotional spectrum. All premeds and future physicians employ a steely determination, an unwillingness to flinch in the face of difficult situations. In undergrad, med school, residency, and beyond, trainees "do one" on a daily basis, learning new skills at a rapid pace. They eventually reach proficiency and ultimately expertise, allowing them to practice medicine with precision and "teach one" to the generations that follow.

But there is a limitation to this approach to the premedical process, and it lies in the "see one" portion. The vast majority of aspiring premeds have limited exposure to the actual life experience of a career in medicine, at all stages from medical school to residency to practice as a full-fledged physician. This is to no fault of their own, as this vital information is neither easily attainable nor readily accessible. The "see one" step of the premedical process is often stunted, as it is difficult for many premeds to find real clinical experience until they start medical school and begin a structured training program. Perhaps without even knowing it, many aspiring students commit to a tremendously challenging road without the ability to see what they are committing to, without the opportunity to understand what life as a physician is truly like.

Yet medicine is still an exceedingly popular career choice, with one of the most competitive graduate school admissions processes and more than 50,000 students applying to US medical schools each year since 2015[1]. And herein lies the counterintuitive notion which I call *the premed paradox:*

How could so many intelligent and hardworking people dedicate their lives to becoming a physician, perhaps the longest and most arduous professional path, with such little information about what that commitment actually entails?

The farther I have moved along in my medical training and now my career, the more data I have gathered to argue that the premed paradox exists and the more the paradox has continued to perplex me. From what I have seen through my experience, as well as those of my peers and countless students I have mentored, most premeds are affected by the paradox at least to some degree, lacking a level of exposure which would truly prepare them for the career that lies ahead. Ironically, but not surprisingly, I was as much a subject in my own data set as any other individual. Despite the considerable benefit of having a physician as a father, who certainly provided me with great advice as I embarked on a medical career, I still had a relatively elementary understanding of what my future in medicine would actually look like.

I am no exception to the rule—I am a confirmation of it.

Though a medical career is a worthwhile and noble pursuit, it should be chosen carefully with sound motivations. If not, and the individual's expectations are not met, there is a much higher chance for professional dissatisfaction and ultimately burnout.

If, on the other hand, the career choice is aligned with the individual's values based on solid information and experience, a happy and fruitful work life is a much more likely outcome. We all deserve this opportunity for professional gratification. I feel very fortunate that I ultimately found it. With the right knowledge and exposure, *you* can find it as well.

A few years ago, as I navigated the challenges of my early career, I realized I was passionate about mentoring future physicians and helping them find this crucial knowledge. I felt a desire, even a duty, to empower those who would come after me with the perspective I gained over years of work in the medical field. It became my goal to distill my experiences into an honest and comprehensive picture of the life of a physician, from education to training all the way to a career as a medical doctor. I wanted to empower future physicians with the knowledge they need to understand and appreciate this complex career. This was the best solution I could conjure to combat the premed paradox and to pay it forward to the next generation of physicians.

The result of that effort is this book. Within its pages lies a fund of knowledge which is essential for anyone considering the medical profession. These experiences and anecdotes answer the questions, "What do you wish you knew before you started your career in medicine? What have you learned along the way? What is the experience of a physician truly like?"

These important questions are at the core of my reflections and those of many of my peers in the medical field. In answering them, I hope to prepare others better than I was prepared when I embarked on this journey many years ago.

Chapter 2: Ignorance and Inertia

Today I have the privilege of caring for patients in the hospital, adults who are sick enough to require admission from the emergency room (ER) to a medical ward. I am what we call a "hospitalist"—a physician who works exclusively in the hospital and specializes in the care of a broad range of diseases in hospitalized patients. I completed residency training in internal medicine and elected to pursue hospital medicine, applying my skills to the care of acutely ill patients on various medical floors as well as the intensive care unit (ICU).

I care for patients with a variety of conditions affecting nearly every organ system, from strokes to heart attacks, pneumonia to kidney failure, fractures to intestinal bleeds, cancer to liver failure. As hospitalists, we see it all and there is no lack of variety. Each week I care for a new set of patients with unique medical issues and even more unique social backgrounds and life stories. I love what I do. I have the honor of helping people through tremendously difficult moments in their lives. With that comes a rich but varied emotional experience, with ups and downs, challenges and triumphs on a daily basis.

When I reflect on my path, I aspired to join the medical profession for a number of reasons, many of which were not unlike my peers: intellectual curiosity about the human body; a desire to positively impact the lives of those around me; the lifelong example of my father who was a physician; and the goals of professional satisfaction and financial stability, which I believed medicine could provide. But in addition to these factors, which were certainly strong players, I can't deny two others which are slightly embarrassing to acknowledge today: *ignorance* and *inertia*.

Let's start with the first factor: *ignorance*. Though this term generally carries a negative connotation, I use this word in its most literal sense, absent of its usual baggage. I don't mean to say that I was intentionally ignoring information which was readily available; I was certainly trying to seek insight into the medical field and my potential future career (in other words, "see one"). But at the time, I simply did not know as much as I should have about what medical training and practice would be like. I couldn't fully grasp what it would look like or feel like to be a physician. The details of life as a medical student, resident, and physician felt distant: the hours, the workflow, the feeling of being in a hospital or clinic day in and day out, caring for human lives. It all still felt quite abstract. At that young age, with naturally limited life experience, the true feeling of a career caring for human lives was difficult to fathom. I was trying to grasp it and seek the right information. But if I am being honest in retrospect, I'm not even sure I knew the right questions to ask.

Sure, I had the general idea down: I knew I needed to succeed in my undergraduate studies over the course of four years, followed by a rigorous four years of med school, in turn followed by a challenging residency training which would lead to my career as a physician. But to be frank, I knew very little about what the experience of med school was actually like and even less about what residency training entailed. I definitely did not know how long different residencies (or fellowships) lasted, how many years it might require to reach my goals, and what different types of medical practice or career interests I could pursue once I was done training.

Now, let me be clear: no one has an exact understanding of the steps that lie ahead, the ability to predict each twist and turn along the long road that makes up a career or a lifetime. There is inherent uncertainty in all of our futures. In medicine, law, engineering, finance, entrepreneurship, or any other professional path, most people start with incomplete knowledge of what lies ahead, and things do not always go as planned.

What I do think is important in any career path though, and particularly in the case of medicine, is to have at least a basic understanding of what life in that field will be like. It is invaluable to have a roadmap of medical training, the different career choices available within medicine, and the emotional experiences that come along with it. It is crucial to understand the real-life outcomes of work as a physician, both positive and negative. This knowledge is a must. It is a baseline level of exposure that every aspiring premedical student has a right (and maybe even a responsibility) to know.

Now let's circle back to the second subtle factor which influenced my path toward a career in medicine: *inertia*. Though I was not careless with my choice to pursue a career as a physician, as it was made with a fair amount of thought, there was a certain momentum associated with it: once the tires were rolling downhill, it was very difficult to slow down, dismount, and consider whether I was on the right path in the first place.

There is a certain gravitational pull when it comes to the medical profession that can keep one pushing forth for a decade or more despite difficult odds. Persisting in this manner is somewhat adaptive, as medical training is inherently difficult, requiring patience and perseverance. But I would hope that for all premeds, this pull does not come at the cost of deliberate self-reflection. Commitment to a career as a physician is a wonderful undertaking, but one to be chosen carefully for the right reasons. Through thoughtful reflection on your own values, while seeking the right experience and exposure, you can bolster your resolve and preparation for this amazing career.

While my own career slowly evolved, my passion for medicine grew in parallel with my knowledge and skill. Today, I feel very fortunate to practice this sacred art. It is an honor to heal patients and, perhaps more importantly, support them with empathy and compassion in their most trying moments. But as is true of almost anything in life, there are two sides to the story: with fulfillment and gratification come challenges and adversity. The practice of medicine is a perfect representation of life's balanced duality. In the next chapter, we will explore the dual nature of medicine. In doing so, we will develop a stronger understanding of the nuance and complexity of this remarkable career.

Chapter 3: Duality

In the practice of medicine, we deal with the extremes of life and death. We can treat patients from the brink of death back to solid health. We at times perform miracles, reviving patients not only from near-death but from actual death (more on this in a moment). Despite the incredible outcomes we can achieve in medicine, we do not always win the battle against disease. In fact, in the critically ill patient, we often do not. This is a sobering reality of medicine and life, but one we cannot deny. What we can do as physicians is strive to maintain good health and quality of life for our patients for as long as possible.

There is dichotomy in life and death and there is dichotomy in the practice of medicine. The two sides of this age-old practice are each as relevant today as they were in its most primitive inception. Medicine provides fulfillment—it is a means by which one can touch the lives of others in a uniquely impactful way. But it also serves a healthy dollop of hardship, both in the pursuit of medical expertise and in its day-to-day practice. To ignore this multifaceted nature of medicine would be naïve, perhaps even irresponsible.

With that thought in mind, let's explore the rich duality of physician life. In particular, I would like to recount two vivid memories from my residency training. Though they occurred only weeks apart, they perfectly encapsulate the broad emotional experience that comes with a career as a physician. The two experiences share many similarities in terms of the high-stakes decision making and complex skills they required. Yet they ended in vastly different ways. Taken together, these memories reflect the dichotomy that is a defining feature of medical practice. They are undoubtedly poignant to me, as they were moving moments that are seared in my consciousness. But more than that, they are an opportunity to explore the deep and varied emotional experience of a physician. They are an opportunity to learn and grow together.

I slowly approached the hospital in a dimly lit silence, the streetlamps flickering in the crisp morning air. It was winter, and the sun liked to take its time rising this time of year. I could see my breath swirling in front of me as I walked, the clouds of mist a solitary interruption of the morning darkness. The stroll offered little to stimulate the senses—the city streets were rarely as quiet as they were at this hour. But I enjoyed the silence. The atmosphere allowed for a sort of peaceful escape, even if only for a few moments out of the day.

Inside the hospital was not quiet, that much I knew. Those walls housed more activity than most could imagine, from the raucous emergency room to the bustling operating rooms to the floors full of patients with every malady you could think of. The patients seemed to represent the full spectrum of humanity. They hailed from countless walks of life, but all came for the same purpose: the chance to live, breathe, walk, or talk—the chance to feel just a little better. It was our job as medical professionals to realize those hopes on their behalf.

Today I would be right in the thick of it all, caring for the hospital's sickest patients in the ICU. This shift was just another in a string of weeks and months spent honing my craft as an internal medicine resident. Residency was the time to truly become a physician, to learn what is needed to effectively care for living, breathing patients. We grew accustomed to the daily grind, partly out of necessity and partly because we appreciated how much we were growing in the process.

During rounds that morning, I met a patient who was quite ill but somewhat stable at that point. He was relatively young and healthy with few preexisting medical conditions. He came in overnight for respiratory failure, the cause of which was still unclear. I took over his care that day as the senior medical resident on the ICU team.

Patients can be admitted to the ICU for a multitude of reasons, but most boil down to a few root problems: severe respiratory issues requiring breathing support (such as a ventilator); severe circulatory issues requiring medications to boost the blood pressure; severe kidney issues requiring a specific form of dialysis; severe neurologic issues requiring specialized medications and frequent neurologic monitoring; or any severe medical/surgical issue requiring the highest level of nursing care.

For this patient, his breathing was the primary issue when he was admitted to the hospital. At the time I first encountered the patient though, he was improving from a respiratory standpoint, and I was nearly certain that he wouldn't require a ventilator. But as I have come to find over the years, certainty is almost non-existent when it comes to medical practice. Despite our experience and best predictions, at the end of the day, we never truly know what is going to happen to the patient. That is part of the inherent excitement and challenge of this career.

This case was a testament to that lack of certainty. Despite a fairly routine morning, later in the day, the patient's blood pressure began to drop to an unsafe level. I placed a central venous catheter (a special IV line) in a large vein in the patient's neck, and we began to treat him with medications to keep his blood pressure up as well as antibiotics for a presumed infection. Things were stable for the moment.

Then that evening, somewhat out of the blue, things took a dire turn. The patient's mental status declined significantly, and his breathing became very labored, concerning for impending failure of his lungs. Despite my predictions, the patient eventually had to be intubated and connected to a ventilator to support his breathing. Blood tests showed that his body was producing an extremely high amount of acid, unfit for appropriate function of the vital organs. We placed another central line needed to start dialysis, using a machine to take the place of his kidneys and remove the acid from his blood. As is always the case when a young patient is quickly declining, the stress was mounting. But I felt cautiously optimistic that we would see this patient through, as we had treatments in place for each of his severe medical issues.

Initially, these efforts worked. For a few hours, the patient stabilized again. Such is life in the ICU—with our best impression of our firefighting sisters and brothers, we put out medical fires one-by-one as they arise. Unfortunately, this was not the last fire of the night. The acid in the patient's blood began to rise once again, this time to an even higher level—one not compatible with life.

Concerned for a source of infection or ischemia (lack of blood flow to an organ) which could not be treated with antibiotics and medications alone, we performed scans of much of his body. They showed nothing, no explanation for his severe illness. None of his blood work or cultures could explain the severity of his condition either. Despite such a broad evaluation and discussion among several experienced physicians at this point, there was no clear cause of his decline and no alternative treatment course to pursue. I felt exhausted and hopeless; though I had been practicing long enough to know that in some cases there was no answer to the medical mystery, these moments still cut deep. This was one of those rare situations. Unfortunately, there was nothing more we could do.

By the next morning (at which point I was still on call, nearing the twenty-four-hour mark of my thirty-hour shift), the patient had gone into multi-organ failure. We knew the level of acid in his blood was going to cause cardiac arrest very soon. We had to face the terrible reality that, in this rare case, medicine would not only fail to save his life, but could not even explain why he needed saving in the first place. As a physician, this is a tough pill to swallow.

Perhaps even tougher was seeing the patient's family suffer. I spoke with them throughout the process, updating them on how their father was being treated and what we were hoping to achieve with his care. On that morning, when we knew that the patient would soon pass away, I wiped the fatigue from my eyes and stepped into the room with a heavy heart. I knew that no matter how tired I was, this moment was crucial. I needed to be composed. I needed to be strong for the family.

In medicine we deal with death not infrequently, but it hurts much more when it is so unexpected and inexplicable. I will never forget one of his children's reactions: first with shocked questions, next with violent sobs, and finally by shouting in disbelief. His father had been talking, eating, walking leisurely only days prior. How could he now be at death's doorstep?

These moments are psychologically and emotionally taxing, no matter who you are or how you approach them. I was truly sad for the patient and his family. But somehow in these moments, we must call on an inner resolve, a knowledge that we have a unique responsibility to be strong, to help ease suffering in whatever way we can for the sake of those we care for.

Within two hours of our morning discussion, the patient passed away. It demanded much of my inner strength to remain composed and comfort the family with a steady presence. I tried to empathize but knew that I could not fully fathom the enormity of their loss. The toll on me and my team was considerable, but surely it was nothing compared to what they had to bear. I could only hope that we had helped the patient and his loved ones in some small way during that difficult time.

This is often the only solace we as physicians can take in moments like this: that hopefully we eased the patient's suffering and provided some support to their loved ones during what can only be described as a gut-wrenching process. We must hope that our empathy and compassion provide some comfort through the pain. With that thought in mind, we hold our heads high and we push on. We keep fighting day in and day out, for our patients and their families.

As physicians, we must recognize that these experiences will be part of the process. No matter how excellent the physician or how expert the medical care, sometimes disease will triumph. We must deal with these perceived failures and recognize that sometimes the outcome is out of our hands. Though we do our best and fight for our patients, we must be ready to accept death and loss. By recognizing this, we are better prepared for life as a physician. We can build strategies to cope—whether it be sharing the challenging experience with a trusted colleague or friend, taking a moment to pay respect to the life of a lost patient, or using the experience to learn and grow amidst the pain. Understanding the inevitability of these experiences is an important step for physicians and aspiring premeds alike.

Later that same month, in the middle of the night, I was awoken from a deep (albeit brief) slumber. The ring of my pager pierced the silence. I was all too familiar with that sound. *Maybe familiarity is finally breeding contempt,* I chuckled while lying in the call room bed. My eyes struggled to open, as if their lids were bogged down by an invisible weight. I stretched my hand to the bedside table. As quickly as I could, I wiped the sleep from my eyes and focused on the pager that had ended my early-morning siesta. It was 3:00 AM, and a nurse on the seventh floor needed me.

I was the ICU resident on-call, once again on a thirty-hour shift, and had completed about twenty hours so far. It was rare that I slept at all on these shifts; so as much as it pained me to rise from the warmth of the bed, I had to count my blessings that I was able to catch at least a quick bit of rest.

As I was sliding on my shoes and heading over to the phone to give the nurse a call, I was accosted by another, even less inviting sound. The hospital PA system rang out loudly "Code Blue, Seven West. Code Blue, Seven West." *Same unit,* I thought. *Must be the same patient...Alright, here we go. It's go time!*

This overhead "code blue" call is never a welcome noise for any healthcare worker in the hospital, as it signifies that a patient has suffered a cardiac arrest and requires cardiopulmonary resuscitation (CPR). As the senior resident in the ICU that night, I was responsible for running this code: it was my job to find this patient as fast as possible and lead a medical team's effort to save the patient's life. With this opportunity comes a surge of anxiety, as is unavoidable when the stakes are as high as life and death. But it also brings the excitement which comes with an amazing chance to make a real difference—to truly save a patient's life.

When we revive a patient with CPR during a code blue situation, we are doing so because the patient's heart has stopped beating and their lungs have stopped breathing. This means that, by definition, the patient has died, and we are literally attempting to bring them back to life. The goal of the code blue is to restore the heart's inherent rhythm and maintain blood flow to the body's organs. CPR consists of a combination of chest compressions, medications, and sometime electric shocks. By physically compressing the heart with our hands through the chest wall (because the heart is no longer beating on its own), we can help the heart eject blood through the aorta, supplying the organs with the oxygen needed to maintain life. We also provide medications such as epinephrine which can boost the blood pressure and increase blood flow. If enough blood is circulated back to the heart itself, the heart can eventually reinitiate its own inherent rhythm. Put simply, we can kickstart the body's engine after it has stalled. In some situations, electric shocks are needed to convert the heart from an unstable rhythm to a normal one, thereby restoring its inherent pumping function. All the while, we provide breaths to the patient, first with a mask and bag filled with oxygen and then by use of a ventilator. This supplies oxygen to the blood as it circulates to the vital organs. Finally, we determine and correct the underlying cause of the cardiac arrest, whether it be a disturbance in blood electrolytes, low blood oxygen, bleeding, infection, and so on.

A code blue is controlled chaos. Several medical professionals are in the room each performing a crucial task: nurses (and sometimes medical students or residents) positioning the patient, performing chest compressions, and administering medications; respiratory therapists providing ventilations; an anesthesiologist or critical care physician intubating the patient, connecting them to the ventilator, or obtaining adequate IV access; pharmacists preparing and delivering medications; and a code leader, the physician at the foot of the patient's bed analyzing the situation, making medical decisions, and providing orders to be carried out by the unified team.

Sometimes (but not always), amidst the chaos we achieve the ultimate success: saving the patient's life. Bringing patients back from the dead seemed like science fiction to me when I first encountered this concept in medical school, but it is a real part of medical practice. This was an amazing realization when I grasped it in those literal terms. Experiencing a successful code blue is nothing short of extraordinary. The feeling of excitement and adrenaline, success mixed with relief, is incredible. Eventually watching the patient recover and leave the hospital is extremely rewarding. This is an exhilarating experience, a privilege unique to the practice of medicine.

There was a time when running a code blue would have been terrifying for me. But with effort and experience comes skill and steadiness. Though resuscitating a patient is never easy, I knew what I was heading into. I knew I could do it. I had done it before, after all, and I trusted my training to serve me now when I needed it once again.

When I arrived at the patient's bedside, I quickly surveyed the scene. I identified myself to the code nurse as the code leader, so that we could keep a clear stream of communication as we directed the team. The patient's primary nurse began quickly providing me a report of his previous condition and the events leading up to the cardiac arrest. I synthesized the info as quickly as possible while my eyes scanned the room, assessing where we stood and what needed to be done.

Keeping a cool head and clear mind is crucial as the code leader. I took a few deep breaths to steady myself. Chest compressions were underway, taking the place of the heartbeat and supplying blood to the patient's organs. I began to call out orders, including epinephrine to be delivered to the patient in an effort to get the blood pressure up and the heart going once again. The anesthesiologist had arrived and was working on placing a breathing tube down the patient's throat, which would allow us to deliver oxygen via the ventilator. Things were going appropriately up there, so I directed my attention to the next several tasks. We secured effective IV access by placing an interosseus IV line. This is a line which goes directly into the patient's bone, allowing us to quickly administer crucial medications. It sounds brutal, but it can be a necessary measure to save the patient's life.

Meanwhile, we needed to analyze the patient's heart rhythm via a cardiac monitor. I called for the rhythm analysis and took a quick look, recalling my training as I read. It was a rhythm called ventricular fibrillation, which is a common cause of cardiac arrest. Due to inadequate electrical activity, the heart's larger chambers (the ventricles) quiver rather than pumping in a synchronous fashion. This rhythm is one that is best treated by electrical shocks in addition to IV medications.

Many of us recall medical shows or movies in which the physician calls "CLEAR" and an electrical shock is delivered to the patient. The purpose of calling "CLEAR" is to make sure everyone is cleared from touching the patient, so that the electrical current is not transmitted to others who are providing care. The shock can be painful, but it is a potentially life-saving intervention.

We prepared the defibrillator—a machine which allows for delivery of an electrical shock when needed—and attached it to the patient. Once charged, I called "CLEAR" as I surveyed those around me to ensure that, just for a moment, no one was touching the patient. I then pressed the large red button and delivered the shock, a jolt of electricity running through the patient's body. As soon as this was done, those delivering chest compressions and breaths moved right back into place. It is crucial not to interrupt breaths and compressions for long during a code, as these are the interventions which supply oxygen to the blood and blood to the body.

Next, some of the patient's immediate blood work began to return. We found that his potassium was far too high, which is a strong risk factor for developing a dangerous heart rhythm. We quickly delivered IV medications which reduce the level of potassium in the blood and stabilize the heart. More blood work showed that the patient's pH was low, meaning his body was producing a high amount of acid, which is a common consequence of inadequate blood flow to the organs. We provided more IV medications to neutralize the acid and restore a safer blood pH. Finally, we continued to administer epinephrine, our strongest method to augment the blood pressure and continue the circulation of blood throughout the body. Through these efforts, we were not only attempting to restore the heart's innate rhythm, but also address the underlying causes which may have incited the issue in the first place.

My mind quickly raced as I went down my mental checklist, the crucial to-dos of a code blue. If I could deliver on these tasks effectively in conjunction with the coordinated medical team, we might be able to save this patient's life. It was time to analyze the rhythm once again. Still in ventricular fibrillation, the patient needed another shock. Another round of charging the machine and calling "CLEAR," and an electrical current was again delivered to the patient's chest just over the heart. This time, I held my breath as we checked the rhythm. It appeared that it had returned to normal, that the patient's heart was pumping correctly with the appropriate electrical current. We quickly checked the patient for a pulse.

"I have a pulse," yelled one of the nurses at the patient's bedside, hand on the femoral artery in the groin. "I HAVE A PULSE!"

Yes! I thought to myself. *Almost there!* As the patient's heart was once again pumping on its own, we paused our chest compressions. We checked the blood pressure and found that the patient was stabilizing. We call this a "return of spontaneous circulation," meaning that the patient's heart is pumping on its own once again and blood flow has been restored to at least a reasonably safe level. The patient was maintaining his blood pressure adequately and the heart was pumping appropriately.

YES! WE DID IT! My mind raced as I celebrated this positive outcome. I was excited and relieved, but the challenges certainly did not end there. I knew how much more we had to do. Even after the heart is pumping again on its own and the code blue is completed successfully, the patient must fight a difficult battle in the ICU. We transferred the patient and cared for him diligently over the next couple of weeks. He was monitored closely by countless members of the team; eventually he was able to be weaned off the ventilator and breathe on his own once again. Next, he slowly regained the strength needed to stand up and walk across the room. These seemingly small steps are monumental achievements when you nearly lost your life. But the patient battled, as did we on his medical team, and together we were able to see it through. He eventually made a full recovery and was able to return home.

This was a medical triumph I will always remember. It certainly was not mine to claim alone; numerous medical providers worked with me the night of the cardiac arrest and throughout the patient's long stay in the ICU. The patient himself showed tremendous strength to persevere and recover as he did. His family supported him every step of the way, providing the love that inspires such strength. It was an absolute team effort. But I could not help but feel the personal fulfillment that comes with caring for a patient in such a powerful way, of helping redirect the path of someone's life. I will never forget the experience.

Moments like this are the grand gestures that medicine makes, reminding us how fulfilling the career can be. But just as important are the simple daily moments: taking the extra time to listen to a patient struggling with depression; extending a hand of compassion to the patient who just received a cancer diagnosis; making sure to answer all the questions of a young couple struggling with infertility. These simple moments of compassion and empathy, coupled with the grand, life-saving moments that come along every so often, make the practice of medicine truly special. They have fueled my passion for this career. They have confirmed to me that no matter how challenging it is, life as a physician is an incredible privilege.

Just like the previous story with a negative patient outcome, this positive experience will stay with me forever. It is critical to my identity as a physician because it represents the successes and highs that also will come with a medical career. Often the toughest moments are countered by the positive ones, the triumphs which lead the patient back to health and happiness. This balance helps restore equilibrium to the daily tumult of medical life. These unique professional experiences are ones you can only have in the practice of medicine—they cannot be reproduced elsewhere. They are moments which can move you in ways you did not think possible. I believe that this duality, this broad and deep emotional experience, is what is most compelling about the practice of medicine.

And thus, we return to the core reason I endeavored to write this book: to empower future generations of physicians with exposure to the full spectrum of experience within a career in medicine, so that they may be as informed as possible when they embark upon their own professional path. Through these pages, the countless talented and noble individuals who aspire to a career in medicine will gain the knowledge they need to approach it with confidence. For others not directly within the medical field, this book will provide a unique perspective on the life of a medical student, resident, and physician, illuminating an otherwise nebulous but exciting world. We will take an in-depth look at what life as a physician is truly like. Along the way we will address the key components of medical education, training, and career practice, and how they lead to the actual *experience* of a physician. And this will be our true focus—not how to get into medical school or the steps necessary to become a medical doctor; while important, there are countless existing resources which tackle these topics effectively. Rather, we will dive deep into a more poorly described concept: *the comprehensive physician experience,* and what that means for a life in medicine.

Part II: Preparation

Chapter 4: Why Medicine?

Medicine is a dynamic field in so many ways, but two particularly important ones are its breadth and diversity. In a sense, there is something for everyone in medical practice, if only they search hard enough. Though the field itself is a community of driven and relatively like-minded individuals, it also is composed of a broad array of specialties, practice settings, and career choices which allow for a huge diversity of interests. We will delve into those nuances more in chapters to come. But here is why I bring them up now: this diversity of experience is a key feature of medicine that is one of its biggest strengths as a career path. In the same way that it provides a broad array of opportunities, medicine attracts a diverse range of people who pursue it for a multitude of reasons. Though there are certainly some common reasons why people choose to pursue a career as a physician, many of which we will touch on shortly, no two individuals have the exact same experience which leads them to the field.

In fact, it is unlikely that any individual has one sole reason why they want to become a doctor. A choice as profound as becoming a physician is typically based on multiple reasons. It is best if each reason is well-developed and well-explored. Just like choosing a life partner, pursuing medicine greatly alters the arc of one's life. Though some may believe in love at first sight, most would cite a number of reasons why they love their partner and several characteristics which make them a good match. Beauty or an instantaneous attraction is seldom enough to maintain a happy, lifelong relationship. A career choice, medicine in particular, is no different.

To each and every person who chooses to pursue a career as a physician, I offer my congratulations and my heartfelt welcome. It is only my desire that before doing so, you allow yourself the necessary time for self-reflection. Though you will be asked in medical school (and residency) interviews why you want to become a physician, there is no "correct" answer. Arriving at the decision is a personal process that we all experience differently. Consequently, I can't tell you why to pursue medicine or how to determine if it is truly right for you. What I can tell you is this: whatever your current notions of why you want to become a physician are, and however sure you are, you should evaluate them carefully. This is a decision to be made with considerable thought and introspection, and now is the perfect opportunity to start that process.

Start with Self-Reflection

Start by thinking deeply about yourself. Reflect on your strengths and weaknesses, your interests, your personal and professional goals. All these factors play a role in determining what career is right for you. The key is to not be a passive actor, not to allow inertia to keep you on a path which may not be the best one for you. Throughout this book, try to actively engage with the content. As you read, think about your own priorities, goals, and where you want to see yourself in the future. This is the perfect time to perform that necessary self-reflection. I can assure you that by doing so, you will be better prepared to pursue your future career. In performing this exercise, you will uncover and better understand your own reasons for choosing the path to becoming a physician.

There are many reasons, of varying degrees of quality, for pursuing a career in medicine. Let's walk through the most common reasons one-by-one and critically evaluate each. Some of them may be your own reasons and some may be ones you have not thought about. In considering these reasons, you can understand the vast motivations for pursuing medicine, and lay the framework of your own professional goals along the way.

Why Did Most Physicians Choose this Career Path?

When evaluating the top reasons to pursue a career as a physician, why not take a lesson from the generations who have come before? While considering any career, asking for perspective from those who have already walked the path is a great place to start.

Luckily, I have already asked for you! After reflecting on my personal experiences, those of my peers, and my time mentoring dozens of premeds and medical students, I distilled the several repeated reasons to pursue a career as a physician. Here are the most common reasons, discussed point-by-point and graded on a scale of strength. Imagine these points as possible building blocks for the house that will be your future medical career. I will consider each block here and rate its ability to serve as a sound component of your foundation. I will use the following four designations of quality, from best to worst, to help you gauge how sound these reasons are: *great*, *good*, *mediocre*, and of course, *bad*.

1. **I want to help people** – *Great, but not enough...*

This is probably the most commonly cited reason to pursue a career in medicine. Though it has in some ways reached cliché status, that does not necessarily make it a bad reason. In fact, I would consider it a great reason to pursue medicine. But in and of itself, this is not enough. One should have multiple additional reasons, strong and sound, to carry them through the challenges of a career in medicine.

Though it is not unique, I do think this reason is quite important. In a way, it should almost be a prerequisite, something that any future physician should feel in some way. Most of our lives in medicine are spent in the service of others in need; therefore, a desire to help others is perfectly suited to a career as a physician. But there are countless other professionals who provide important help to others: from the accountant who prepares taxes (I thank mine profusely each year for providing me peace of mind), to the engineer who designs iPads (a friend of mine does this and I would say it is a huge help to the daily lives of many people), to the chef who fills the bellies of joyous customers (if great food doesn't make the world a better place, I don't know what does). Though essential and necessary to a rewarding career as a physician, a desire to help people is not specific to the path. Alone, it is unlikely to be enough.

2. **I am interested in the human body (anatomy, physiology, etc.)** – *Great*

This is what I would consider another near prerequisite for a fruitful career in medicine. There is no denying that medical education is grueling. Though I will share some secrets within these pages, this is not one of them. But work can become play when genuine interest is involved. I truly enjoyed learning about cardiac and pulmonary physiology in college, medical school, and beyond. I still remember my first encounter with these concepts in a physiology course during undergrad at

UCLA. I was excited to say the least. This interest fueled my already budding desire to pursue medicine. It is important to have that interest going into medical school, as it makes learning enjoyable and not simply a chore.

In many ways, gaining knowledge in medical school was a lot of fun. But I will be honest and admit that studying the volumes of information we were expected to master as a medical student was not all fun and games. It was often a grind. That is the reality of it. But having the foundation of a genuine interest in the human body will make the process of learning an engaging one, despite the long hours of studying that would be burdensome to anyone. The interest will carry you through those tough years and perhaps become even more important down the line when you need to continue learning in the ever-changing landscape of medical information.

This reason is essential, and if you don't honestly harbor this interest, I would seriously consider whether medicine is the right fit for you.

3. I want to work and interact with people on a daily basis
   – *Great*

This is overall a very solid reason to become a physician. The practice of medicine is absolutely an interpersonal exercise. If you desire a career in which you will meet new people each day and have face-to-face encounters with a multitude of individuals from very diverse walks of life, a career as physician is a great choice. Many think of the most obvious example of this: the doctor-patient encounter. Undoubtedly, as a physician you will have a vast array of social interactions with many patients each day. Some of them will be pleasant and some of them will be challenging (or even down-right contentious), but day-to-day life as a physician will certainly bring human variety. The average physician might see twenty or more patients daily, so a unique and ever-changing interpersonal experience certainly awaits you in this field.

Another aspect of interaction in a physician's career which is more overlooked is the interface with an array of healthcare professionals. When I reflect on my practice as a hospitalist, admitting patients from the ER and caring for them throughout their hospital stay, I can think of dozens of healthcare professionals and other essential workers who I interact with on a daily basis. With each patient I care for there is also a nurse, a nursing assistant, a pharmacist, a social worker and/or case manager, sometimes other consulting physicians (or at least the emergency physician who called me for the admission), often a physical therapist and/or occupational therapist, and the list goes on. I would estimate I easily interact with over fifty healthcare professionals on a typical shift in the hospital, and no two days are the same. Medicine truly is a team sport, of which the patient and physician are the central players.

If this variety of interpersonal interaction interests you, medicine could be a great path. If you prefer more solitary, individual pursuits, perhaps medicine is not the best choice. If you are not particularly fond of this level of social interaction, or even irked by it, perhaps think again.

4. I want to make money – *Bad*

For a number of reasons, this is quite simply a bad motivation for a career in medicine. There is no way to sugar coat it. The unfortunate part is that, though I doubt this is the only motivator for most people pursuing medicine, financial gain is a concept that is eternally linked to a career as a physician. This is rooted in the way the medical profession has been perceived historically. For decades, doctors have been viewed as wealthy, commanding salaries and prestige well above the population median. But herein lies the issue: times have changed, and physician finances are much more complex now. While physicians do make a very respectable salary (certainly enough to live well and provide for their families), there are several financial challenges which also accompany a modern medical career: significant debt, delayed earning due to lengthy training, and malpractice lawsuits, to name a few. The concept that physicians are not typically uber-wealthy is perhaps less familiar to those outside of healthcare, but it is something every potential applicant should know. We will discuss these financial aspects of physician life in detail in Chapter 12.

Perhaps most importantly though, pursuing any career solely to make money is generally a poor motivation. It is a recipe for eventual dissatisfaction. Specific to medicine, this reason becomes particularly weak when considering the amount of hard work and sacrifice required to become a physician, as well as the relative misconceptions regarding physician wealth. A desire to make money is not likely to carry one through the challenging times of a medical career. If this is your sole reason to pursue medicine, you may want to think again.

5. **I want the prestige and respect associated with being a physician** – *Mediocre to Bad*

There is certainly an inherent amount of respect that comes with being a physician; most people recognize the humanity and dedication that doctors employ in their daily effort to better the lives of their patients. With that said, a desire for prestige is not a good motivator for a career in medicine because it focuses on external expectations out of one's own control (public perception), rather than inherent fulfillment which the career provides. External motivators of perceived happiness are unlikely to deliver the expected reward in the long run. Intellectual interest in medicine (see number two) and a genuine desire to help others (see number one) are examples of sustainable intrinsic motivators of a happy career.

Medicine also lacks some of the luster it once had. I do admit that being a physician comes with a certain respect from society, and I appreciate and value that recognition. But often physicians are confronted with the uncomfortable truth that patients may not always act with the respect (or even civility) that we expect a doctor to receive. Trust in the medical establishment is not what it once was. In the era of social media and online content, many patients think they know as much or more than their provider and have an unfavorable view of the medical community. Circulating misinformation online also can have a detrimental effect on the physician-patient relationship. The COVID-19 pandemic and significant amounts of misinformation about vaccines and potential treatments (such as ivermectin) are prime examples.

During your career as a physician, you will undoubtedly endure abuse and mistreatment. You will also have triumphant moments when you help patients in profound ways, receiving genuine gratitude and kindness in return. Just be ready to take the good with the bad and know that it is not all glamor and prestige when it comes to the practice of medicine. To be a good physician, you must roll up your sleeves and get in the trenches, experiencing good, bad, and ugly along the way. It is a rich experience, but certainly not an easy path of adoration and acclaim.

6. I want the intellectual stimulation of medical education and practice – *Great*

This motivation is at the heart of a career in medicine and captures one of its most important components: intellectual challenge and stimulation. Over the course of four years of medical school and as many as eight years of residency/fellowship training (depending on the field you choose), medicine is filled with constant learning. As I can attest to now, even after completing medical training and going into career practice, you will surely learn something new each day. Furthermore, medicine is filled with complex decision-making and problem solving each day. Though certain disorders present with typical symptoms and have algorithmic treatment plans, complex cases with multiple medical issues and difficult treatment decisions are commonplace. Often medical diagnoses are not totally clear, and the correct answer must be searched for carefully; meanwhile, treatments require the physician to weigh risks and benefits to arrive at a best course of action. These situations require critical thinking, problem-solving, and swift decision making. If you seek ongoing intellectual challenges, and thrive in such situations, a career as a physician would be a good fit for you.

7. I want to be a lifelong learner – *Great*

As previously alluded to, the body of medical knowledge is both vast and dynamic. Thus, true medical mastery is never attainable, and we are all lifelong learners in medicine. In order to maintain knowledge and clinical acumen, as well as keep up with ever-changing diagnosis and treatment guidelines, we must all continue to read and learn throughout our careers. In some ways, this makes medicine more fun, but it certainly makes it more challenging as well. One microcosm of this is that in each medical specialty, physicians must repeat their standardized exams to maintain board certification typically every ten years. These exams keep physicians up to date on changes in the medical literature. While important, there is no doubt that this obligation can be a thorn in the side of the practicing physician. You don't need to study as much during your career as you do in medical school or residency, but learning is a constant in the life of a physician. If hitting the books or reading to maintain knowledge are simply a chore and never a pleasure, medicine may not be the best fit.

8. I want to do medical research – *Mediocre to Good*

Medical research is certainly a huge part of the healthcare field, and you will interface with it throughout a career as a physician. The vast majority of undergraduates applying to medical school complete medical research to bolster their application. Many continue it throughout med school for the same reasons when it comes to residency applications. Finally, some physicians will pursue a career in research, either alongside clinical practice or as a sole professional focus.

Therefore, a desire to perform medical research is a decent motivation for pursuing a career as a physician. The reason I do not call it a good motivation is that there are other, more direct avenues to a career in medical research. If you genuinely want to spend your time on the research bench and in the lab, or even working with data in clinical research, you might consider a graduate degree such as a master's or PhD. Pursuing an MD-PhD is certainly an option (more on this later) which provides the benefit of medical education/clinical experience to augment your perspective during a career in research. Although a research career by way of med school is a viable and noble path, medical education and residency training require at a minimum seven years and sometimes much longer depending on the specialty (not to mention an additional four or more years for those who chose the MD-PhD degree). If you aspire to focus solely on research and don't think medical training is essential to your future success, consider whether pursuing a more direct path to a research career may be a more worthwhile investment of your time (and money).

9. I have a personal or family experience with medicine/illness that drives me to pursue it – *Good*

Overall, this is a good reason to pursue medicine if coupled with other genuine motivators that can sustain a career-long interest in medical practice. I myself began to consider medicine in earnest after my own brush with a medical issue. At age fifteen, I tore my anterior cruciate ligament (ACL, a ligament in the knee) while playing competitive basketball. At the time, my whole life was basketball, or so it seemed. I missed my entire junior year of varsity basketball, undergoing surgery and an eight-month physical rehabilitation process. With the help of my surgeon and dedicated physical therapists, I was able to regain my health and return to the court to play the game I love. This filled a huge void and restored a lot of happiness to my life. The experience allowed me to personally appreciate the immense healing power of medical care.

Many people may have similar and perhaps much more profound or life-altering experiences which drive them toward a career in medicine. Choosing medicine with this motivation is both reasonable and sensible. However, the individual should also have some of the other key components which sustain long term happiness in medicine, ideally an intellectual interest in the study of the human body and its function.

10. I want to serve underserved communities and those in need – *Good*

This in and of itself is a noble motivation to pursue any profession, medicine included. Essentially all medical practice is done in service of those in need; but this is especially pronounced if you choose to practice in areas caring for underserved communities, such as an urban county hospital or a rural medical clinic. A medical career does create a unique skillset and an ability to provide impactful assistance to communities in need. I find this one of the most unique and rewarding components of being a physician.

As mentioned with prior points though, this reason does not reach the *great* designation because it likely needs to be paired with another essential motivator such as an intellectual interest in medicine. You may notice a developing theme here:

certain drivers of medical career interest, though noble and commendable, could be fulfilled with other careers perhaps more easily or sustainably. Therefore, only if coupled with intellectual interest in medicine and lifelong learning do these reasons become *great* motivations for a career as a physician.

11. I do not want a desk job – *Mediocre*

This, in its essence, is a mediocre (to possibly bad) reason to pursue medicine because it is largely based on a misconception: the notion that most jobs require a nine to five schedule of being stationary at a desk and not being out in the field taking action. While many would prefer a more active and dynamic profession, medicine is not necessarily the answer. There are many careers which may afford more flexibility in this regard when taking into account meetings, travel, field work, and the ever-changing prevalence of working from home. Furthermore, much of a career as a physician *is* actually spent at a desk. Why? One simple reason: documentation.

In medicine, note-writing, documentation, and billing (though necessary) have become burdensome. Data suggest that around fifty percent of a physician's time may be spent on the electronic health record (EHR), rather than at the bedside with the patient[1,2]. Though this varies by specialty and individual provider, all physicians spend a considerable portion of their time on the computer. This is unfortunately unavoidable. This phenomenon is a byproduct of a couple of factors. First is the transition to EHRs, which has occurred over the last few decades; though EHRs are instrumental to the accurate, complete, and secure transmission of patient information, there is no denying that they place a large burden of time on the physician to create effective documentation. Second is the manner in which reimbursement for care occurs: billing insurance companies, Medicare, or Medicaid. Billing is predicated on adequate documentation of care provided as well as accurate bill submission. Because of these factors, a significant portion of what physicians do nowadays occurs on the computer and not at the bedside with the patient.

This component of medicine is not glamorous and is certainly not what the aspiring premed envisions when dreaming of becoming a doctor. But it is a doctor's reality, and I would be misleading you if I ignored it. Physicians certainly spend a large amount of time with patients, talking, examining, doing procedures, and providing counseling/support. But they also spend a lot of time sitting at a desk and working on a computer. This is a fact of medical life; for better or for worse, it is here to stay.

12. I want to use my hands and do tangible work – *Good*

This is a reasonable motivation to pursue a career as a physician. It is not a slam dunk, because there are varying degrees of hands-on and procedural work in different medical specialties and because this could potentially be achieved in other lines of work. But there is no denying that if one pursues a career in surgery, there is perhaps no better way to use one's hands for tangible and rewarding work. The healing touch is also prevalent in most specialties simply through the physical exam, and other medical subspecialties such as cardiology, gastroenterology, pulmonology, interventional radiology, and more provide the opportunity for procedural practice. On average, medicine does deliver on this opportunity. If using your hands for meaningful work is important to you, this is not a bad reason to pursue life as a physician, though other motivations would likely need to augment this one to make medicine a great choice.

13. I want to please my parents or impress my family – *Bad*

A desire to please others is flat-out a bad reason to pursue medicine or any other career for that matter. In the case of medicine, a career for which the training requires great determination through years of hard work, a lack of internal motivation will very likely lead to unhappiness and perhaps inadequate performance. I always recommend that those I mentor search inside themselves for what their own true interests and motivations are; without these factors, any career may be a risky choice. Choosing medicine to satisfy external expectations would be a particularly poor decision, as it will come at the cost of (many) thousands of dollars and years of hard work and sacrifice.

14. I want to follow in the footsteps of parents or family – *Mediocre to Good*

Much in the same vein as number thirteen above, this focuses on an external rather than an internal motivator and is therefore at best a good (not great) reason to pursue a career as a physician. It is not uncommon to have had exposure to a parent or family member working in the medical field. This exposure can grow into an interest in the medicine, which can lead to a fruitful career. There is nothing atypical or wrong about this circumstance. My only caution would be to ensure that following in someone else's footsteps only occurs because you truly want to put those shoes on and walk that path yourself. Do not let the experience of others dictate your life choices by virtue of pressure or obligation. If you are fortunate enough, as I was, to have exposure to someone in the medical field, use that as a snapshot of the career that can help you gain insight on whether it is the right fit *for you*. But this is the key: the decision should be about what is right for you and not anyone else.

15. I have already started as premed and don't want to change paths – *Bad*

This reason connects back to the key concept discussed in Chapter 2, a no-no when it comes to determining your future career: inertia. As we understand from Newton's first law, an object in motion stays in motion and an object at rest stays at rest unless acted on by an outside force[3]. When it comes to decisions regarding your career and future, *you* must be that outside force. Do not let the weight of time already spent on an existing path push you further towards something that is not right for you. Before moving any further, take the time to critically reflect. Ask yourself, *Is this really right for me? Is this what I want?*

As I mentioned before, I was as guilty as many when it comes to decision-making inertia, confirming Newton's brilliance just as the physical universe does. Fortunately, I was later able to reflect and I did ultimately find that medicine was a good fit for me. Sometimes I wonder, what if I had not been so fortunate? What if I had chosen poorly and continued moving, inert, down the path of least resistance? Ultimately, I would have met more resistance down the line with the realization that I was less than happy in my career pursuits.

Do not allow yourself to be a casualty of this phenomenon. There is no shame in changing paths. In fact, it is admirable when someone has the bravery to be honest with themself and redirect, still applying dedication and determination to something else that is a better fit for them.

Use this book and each time you gain knowledge (about any field, not just medicine) as an opportunity to challenge the inertia of your existing path. If each time you reflect, you confirm that you are on the right path, you will only be more resolute and more successful in the pursuit of your dreams.

Chapter 5: Is Medicine Right for Me?

Now that we have considered the most common reasons to pursue a career in medicine and critically evaluated each, it's time to get personal. What do I mean by that? It is time to act on the first piece of advice in Chapter 4: begin your self-reflection. Ask yourself the following: as I consider a career in the dynamic field of medicine, how do I evaluate if it is the right choice for me?

There is no formula or secret method to determine this (or any other major life decision for that matter). But there are a number of steps that can help you make meaningful progress in your evaluation of a career as a physician. I outline this method early in the book so that those who need to can actively perform these steps while reading subsequent chapters. Luckily, some of the components of evaluating medicine, particularly gathering information and exposure to the actual experience of medical practice, will be achieved simply by reading this text.

There will be some overlap between the concepts in Chapters 4 and 5, but I outline this approach to serve as an explicit, step-by-step process for considering your potential career in medicine. This deliberate approach will be useful for those who have struggled to find a structured way to evaluate this all-important decision. If you have already made a resolute determination that you will pursue a career as a physician, or if you are already on the path as a medical student or beyond, feel free to skip forward to subsequent chapters. This framework may still be a useful exercise in self-reflection or a reminder about the reasons you love medicine and the motivators that drove you to pursue it. But if it is not necessary for you, by all means, consider moving forward. This book is a tool—use it to serve and guide you in whatever way you need!

A Step-by-Step Framework to Evaluate Your Potential Career in Medicine

1. Gather information.

As with any other decision-making process, first you must do your research. When thinking about a career in medicine, this can be tougher than a simple google search for literature relevant to the topic of a class paper. The internet is certainly a strong place to start, with countless resources about the process of applying to medical school and how to optimize your chances of acceptance. What I have found, though, is that despite the numerous sources helping premeds figure out how to get in, there is a dearth of resources tailored toward teaching them about the actual experience of medical practice. Some good resources do exist; but few websites, videos, or blogs are created for the sole purpose of educating you about what it *feels like* to become a physician and practice as one. Providing the audience this critical information is just as important, if not more important, as it empowers them to decide whether they want to pursue medicine and to attack it with purpose once they have.

You are already taking a huge step toward informing yourself by reading this book. Continue to seek resources which discuss key experiences such as learning in medical school, taking board exams, training during residency, and caring for patients as an attending physician. (An attending is a physician who has completed all medical education/training and now cares for patients independently without supervision). Of course, do not disregard the resources guiding you through study skills, prerequisite courses, exam prep, and applications as these are also very important. But use the experiential resources to augment your understanding of a future life as a physician, rather than simply focusing on how to get there.

Another invaluable resource is direct contact with those who have done it before. For many individuals, it may be logistically challenging to interface with a practicing physician, or even get in contact with one in the first place. If you have an avenue to create this connection, I encourage you to pursue it. Don't be shy. Be mindful and respectful of the physician's time but advocate for yourself so that you may benefit from their experience. Pick the physician's brain about their motivations for pursuing the field as well as their feelings regarding their career experience.

You may recall that as I reflected on my path to my current career, I realized I didn't always know the right questions to ask along the way. Here are some key questions to consider if given the opportunity to discuss a medical career with a physician:

1. What motivated you to become a physician?
2. What do you know now that you wish you knew when you started your journey?
3. What is most rewarding to you in your career?

4. What is most challenging to you in your career? What do you dislike about it?
5. What is the most exciting component of your job?
6. How do you find work-life balance? What sort of time does your career afford to do other things that might be important to you (time with family, other hobbies, etc.)?
7. Do you find your career sustainable? Are you experiencing any burnout, and if so, how do you deal with it/mitigate it? (Burnout is a form of work-related stress, which we will cover in detail in Chapter 15).
8. Did you consider any other careers? What was it about medicine that made it your ultimate choice?
9. In your view, what is the biggest challenge that faces physicians in the future of healthcare?
10. Any specific advice for a premed student considering the path, to help them better understand this important life decision?

Not all of these questions need to be asked; but if given the opportunity, consider these concepts as discussion points that will improve your understanding of the life experience of a physician. For those who are unable to easily make this connection (likely many aspiring premed students), fear not. You can still develop a mature understanding of the medical field with the right resources. Seek sources with honest, unfiltered information about physician life, such as "day in the life" videos or personal accounts of a doctor's experience. These will help you realistically envision a future career as a medical doctor. Direct mentorship is another great avenue for genuine insight and exposure (more on this this to come shortly).

2. **Evaluate your intellectual interests.**
This next step is both critical and simple. You must honestly evaluate whether you harbor an intellectual interest in the study of the human body. This will hopefully become clear with prerequisite courses in undergrad such as anatomy, physiology, or human biology. As you may recall from the prior chapter, this intellectual interest is perhaps the most important reason to pursue a career in medicine, and really should accompany the other reasons if one is to truly enjoy a career as a physician.

Now, let me be honest here: I think most physicians would be lying if they said that they loved every aspect of learning about the human body. We would be misleading you if we said it was always fun, that studying human anatomy or physiology was never a struggle. Studying hard for hours on end, with the pressure of both delivering grades and mastering material, is taxing and can be unpleasant at times. So do not be misled into thinking that you must love every moment of it.

Rather, what is important is the overarching theme of your studies: hopefully you are interested and engaged when learning about the human body. You should have this interest if you are going to succeed in medicine. Without it, the thousands of hours spent studying (yes, I am not exaggerating) in college and medical school will be a burden. If you harbor a true interest in medicine, then learning about human anatomy, physiology, pathology, and medical treatments will be an exciting process. Gaining an understanding and mastery of concepts which were previously hidden from you will be fun. Dissecting the chambers of the heart in anatomy lab, understanding the pathophysiology that drives neurologic disorders like Parkinson's disease, grasping the microbiologic causes of historical diseases like the Plague—these were all exhilarating moments in medical school which I remember clearly. Why? Because I truly enjoyed learning about medicine. Amidst the trials and tribulations of years of training, you will find excitement and fulfillment if you have a genuine intellectual interest human biology.

3. **Evaluate your interpersonal interests.**

Next, take time to evaluate your interpersonal interests. What do I mean by this? Primarily, I recommend considering what type of interpersonal interactions make you happy and excited versus uneasy or uncomfortable. What sort of daily interaction do you see yourself engaging in during your future career? Do you feel more intrigued or anxious about the opportunity to meet and speak (sometimes intimately) with people of all different walks of life each day that you work?

The main point here is to ensure that you are comfortable with the notion of dealing with diverse people with a variety of needs that you will serve to the best of your ability. To many, this variety of interpersonal interaction is what makes medicine most fun. To others, it may be a reason to avoid medical practice altogether. As mentioned before, each patient encounter provides the possibility for great positivity as well as great challenge, perhaps even stress and negativity. The total effect of these encounters can take a toll on the physician over time. But it is my belief that as long as one keeps fighting for their patients and doing what is right, the net outcome of these innumerable doctor-patient encounters will be positive. The patients, after all, are what give our jobs meaning and what make the practice of medicine rewarding.

Just remember that there will always be both good and bad interactions in any job in which you interface with the outside world. As we all know, no job is perfect. As long as you are ready for a great number of interactions with a variety of people, medicine will be a solid choice for you.

4. **Evaluate your personal goals and priorities.**

Once you have evaluated number two and number three above, which I consider to be the most important prerequisites to a successful match with medicine, you should take a close look at your personal priorities and life goals.

Career versus Personal Life

First of all, what is the balance you wish to strike between career and time spent outside of work with family, friends, hobbies, or other pursuits? Though I will not say that medicine and a productive personal life outside the hospital are mutually exclusive, you will certainly have to make some considerable personal sacrifices during your career as a physician. This will be particularly true during medical school and residency/fellowship but will continue to play a role if you opt for a medical specialty which requires overnight, weekend, or holiday work. Specialties which are primarily clinic-based (such as primary care) will in part avoid these schedule challenges as they typically operate Monday through Friday during normal business hours. But even those specialties often require extra work after hours finishing documentation and responding to patient messages, a common challenge in clinic-based medical practice. Essentially all other specialties will have some amount of atypical hours, as most fields have some component of hospital-based work. The hospital never closes, and diseases never sleep. Thus, doctors who work in the hospital will need to be ready for unconventional work hours.

During residency you will often (but not always) work around eighty hours or more per week (twice the typical workweek of forty hours). During this time, you may miss important life moments including weddings, birthdays, and even simply time at home with your family and friends. In a way, this rigor is instrumental to producing medical skill and expertise; but it is undoubtedly taxing. If you prefer a lifestyle that affords you a more conventional schedule, with weekends off and shorter/more predictable hours, other fields may be a better fit. If your highest priority is time spent with loved ones, and you are not willing to sacrifice some of this time for at least seven to ten years through medical school and training, a career as a physician may pose a considerable challenge. I say this not to discourage but to guide: if you are clear and honest with yourself about your goals and priorities now, you may avoid a whole heap of dissatisfaction later. More importantly, you may better realize what sort of career or lifestyle does fit with your goals, which ultimately will improve your career prospects and augment your happiness down the line.

Money and Prestige

I will preface this section by saying that I think neither of these factors should be the primary driver toward any career choice, as discussed in Chapter 4. With that said, it would be foolish to think that for most, they do not play some role in our psyche and how we evaluate the merit of potential professions. We are all human; most of us associate different work with varying levels of inherent value or "prestige." Likewise, no one is immune from considerations of money and the financial implications of a future career. Though it may be more or less important to some of us, we all need money to provide for ourselves and our families. I encourage you to consider now what your financial goals are. In doing so, you may better understand the characteristics of your ideal career choice.

Someone who is likely to be financially satisfied with a career as a physician would have the following characteristics: this individual wants a solid and steady career which will provide the foundation for a secure financial future. They seek a good salary with lower overall job volatility than other industries, and medicine will kindly oblige. This individual is willing to work hard for years, incurring significant debt along the way. They are ready to exercise patience and self-restraint for the first decade or so of their post-undergraduate career as they progress through training toward an attending salary. But they are ok with the waiting game, given the eventual financial reward and security they are likely to capture later in life.

If you are like this individual, you may be very financially satisfied with a career in medicine. If you want to become very wealthy (whatever that means to you) or are seeking early attainment of a high net worth, medicine may not be the best choice. Physicians typically do not attain high amounts of wealth quickly, as medical school is costly and residency/fellowship salaries are modest. The career requires patience and delayed gratification for several years during these stages. Once physicians enter their ultimate career, they are typically good earners, placing them in a strong financial position. But if you want to make millions (of course this is never guaranteed in any field and is much easier said than done), avoid incurring significant debt, and do it all without having to wait years, other lines of work may be a better choice.

Prestige is a trickier entity because it is subjective and depends upon an individual's personal values. I mostly raise this idea because perceived prestige is in some ways a fallacy. Practicing as a physician certainly has inherent value because it helps people, and doctors are therefore recognized for their contributions to society. But to say that it is more or less prestigious than any other profession is risky business (pun intended). Every job, from the postman to the teacher to the CEO of Amazon, has an important role and function in society. No role should be diminished in importance due to perceived prestige as each provides value in some way. Every profession should be respected in its own right.

Furthermore, being a physician may not be as "prestigious" as it is thought to be when you consider that it pays more modestly than most think, demands years of sacrifice, and also requires dealing with difficult treatment from patients, insurance companies, employers, and more. Medicine is a fulfilling and noble field; but its perceived "prestige" may not always amount to what individuals expect.

What I would instead focus on is what *you* value as a worthwhile application of *your own* talents. What would you be excited to do day in and day out? What sort of work would make you proud to call your own? What legacy do you want to leave through your life's work? Identify this, and then strive toward it with passion. Do not focus on what others will think or what you expect the prestige of a career will be. Focus on what you find important, what gives your life meaning, and what brings you personal fulfillment.

5. Get direct exposure.

Alright, take a deep breath. Maybe two. We just covered quite a lot of self-evaluation which is certainly difficult. Confronting these tough questions honestly is no easy task. It is something that can be done over time with careful thought and introspection. But if you have made it through these exercises and feel that medicine is the right fit for you, congratulations! That is a huge step. Now the fun of exploring a career in medicine begins.

The next step in the process is to go beyond evaluating yourself and begin evaluating the career of a physician. Like any other experiment, to conduct an analysis, you first need to gather data. To do so, you must gain direct exposure to the practice of medicine and the reality of becoming a doctor. This step is not always easy and will take some planning and effort on your part. It is absolutely crucial though, because without exposure to components of real medical practice and life, you will be flying blind and choosing a career based on concepts rather than reality.

The three best ways to gain direct exposure to the practice of medicine are the following: volunteer work, shadowing, and research. Each of these activities is an important component of every medical school application, and thus are discussed in many other resources meant to help you get into medical school. But let's think about these steps from an alternative perspective: they are not simply boxes you must check to prove that you have the qualifications to begin your medical training at a respected institution—they are also opportunities to expose yourself to medicine, decide whether you might be happy with the career, and strengthen your understanding of your potential future.

Volunteer work may be the most valuable of the three, as working in a medical setting with some responsibilities may provide you the broadest and most realistic exposure. If possible, seek a position volunteering in a local hospital or medical clinic in any role that interests you. When working, keep your eyes and ears open. Be hard-working and respectful but also be bold. Ask questions (remember those from earlier in this chapter). Utilize the experience to see as much as possible about real life within medicine. It will hopefully be an exciting exploration.

Shadowing, though important, is second in my mind because it can be more of a passive endeavor. It is more directed by the individual being shadowed and can at times be primarily observation and less action. Nevertheless, shadowing can be very helpful as well. What is unique and particularly important to our current cause (critically evaluating a career as a physician), is that it allows you to really put yourself in a doctor's shoes. Most often, shadowing consists of observing a physician's day in a clinic seeing patients. If you are able to shadow in both a clinic and the hospital (and perhaps even in an operating room), the exposure will be even broader. Use this opportunity to get a feel for what daily life as a physician is really like. Imagine yourself in that role and don't be afraid to ask the physician questions regarding their experience. At the same time, keep in mind that this is only a snapshot of medical practice, as there are dozens of specialties and a number of different settings in which doctors can work. Use the experience as a primer but realize that it is not a comprehensive view by any means.

Finally, research experience can help expose you to the actual practice of both clinical and basic science research, which can make up a considerable portion of a career for some physicians. It also will familiarize you with the process of medical discovery and critical thinking/problem-solving. These are skills that physicians use frequently whether in clinical practice or in the research lab. Research is also a great opportunity to again evaluate your intellectual interest in medicine. You don't need to be completely captivated by your research; but hopefully, you will find it engaging to learn more about a specific disease, therapy, organ, or cell. Ideally there will be some spark of interest and some desire to continue expanding your medical knowledge.

By using these three opportunities—volunteering, shadowing, and research—you can perform the data collection and analysis required to answer your own research question: can I see myself being happy as a practicing physician?

6. Seek mentorship.

While obtaining the necessary exposure to a career as a physician, you should also seek guidance and advice. Finding a true mentor through the premed process can be instrumental. In my experience, two types of mentors are most useful. First is someone who may not be much older than yourself who has gone through the process of applying to medical school and/or residency somewhat recently. This may be a medical student, resident, fellow, or even a young attending. The benefit of having this individual's guidance is that they can realistically walk you through what it takes to *become* a physician, having completed some or all of those steps quite recently. Having this perspective will help you understand whether you are willing to do what it takes to climb the mountain of medical education/training.

Next is a more seasoned physician mentor, someone who has completed medical training and is now in practice. This mentorship can be harder to find, as not everyone has a clear path to establishing a connection with a practicing physician. You may have the good fortune of having a personal connection to someone in the medical field, which can be helpful when searching for a mentor. If not, don't be discouraged. Through the avenues of exposure described above (volunteering, shadowing, and research), you will hopefully be able to find a mentor who can provide you realistic guidance and honest feedback.

For some, it may be relatively straightforward to find a mentor. Perhaps you have a family friend who is a physician or know a student who started medical school recently and can show you the ropes. Perhaps you have started a research or clinical volunteering role that provides direct contact with and guidance from medical professionals. But for others, finding a mentor can be a challenge. In addition to avenues already mentioned, consider some of the following strategies to find a personal connection with a mentor in medicine:

1. Professional societies – if you are part of any professional or honors societies, there may be avenues to contact other members who are physicians.

2. Premedical groups/societies – consider joining an on-campus premedical society at your institution. These groups may have networks of contacts or programs which can get you in touch with people working in the medical field.

3. Mentorship programs – some colleges have specific premed mentorship programs. During medical school at UC San Diego, I was part of such a program and was paired with some excellent premed students as their mentor. Sometimes it just takes a deeper investigation of your campus resources to find opportunities like this. You

might benefit from speaking to your academic advisor at the office of your premed major, as they may have experience guiding prior students to the right place for mentorship and exposure.

4. Alumni networks – if you have already graduated college or are part of an alumni network, consider this is a resource to find practicing physicians who might be willing to mentor students.

5. Cold emailing – occasionally being bold and cold emailing a potential mentor can work. For example, a professor who teaches premed students may have knowledge of the medical field or occasionally be an MD themselves. Perhaps they would be willing to be a mentor, or even meet with you occasionally to provide advice.

Keep your eyes open and be creative in your pursuit of information and experience. Don't be afraid to ask questions and advocate for yourself. Hopefully, you will eventually secure a physician mentor who can provide you an honest account of their triumphs and challenges during a career in medicine. The key is to be eager for knowledge but also respectful; if you are able to develop a real connection with this mentor, they will provide you with invaluable perspective. Be curious. Work to understand their experiences, challenges, and successes. In doing so, you may be able to answer some burning questions or tackle the reservations you might harbor about a career as a physician.

7. **Consider alternatives.**

If you have reached this step, you have cleared many hurdles and may be close to or already sure of your career choice. That is excellent progress. Prior to a decision of this magnitude though, it may be prudent to consider potential alternatives.

We have all been asked since our childhood, "What do you want to be when you grow up?" Well now is the time to finally answer that question. Ask yourself, "What might I do if I were to pursue a career other than medicine?" This is an important exercise, and I would guess it is one that most premeds do not perform. In undergrad, I may have daydreamed about a career in basketball (my lifelong obsession) or some other exciting, non-medical field. But in retrospect, I didn't realistically consider alternative career paths when I was a premed pursuing medical school.

When pondering this question, consider some of the same factors discussed previously, including your intellectual interests, interpersonal preferences, and career/personal goals. Are there other career paths which fit your desires as well or better and are realistic/practical to achieve? If so, would you consider them as possible alternative careers? Ultimately, only you can answer this question. Only you know what is best for yourself.

Next comes an important step which I also never performed, which may be overlooked by many. It is reasonable to consider alternative career choices *within* healthcare, as they may offer similar intellectual and interpersonal benefits while avoiding some potential pitfalls of a career as a physician. This is not meant to discourage anyone from becoming a physician or to encourage them to pursue alternative paths. This is only to remind readers that there are many career choices within healthcare, all of which are important and rewarding. Perhaps one of them is a great fit for you and perhaps not. Either way, it is mature and intelligent to be aware of the options within the medical field and to consider them if you are not completely decided on your path as a future physician.

We will cover many of these alternative options in detail in Chapter 7, so stay tuned. For now, suffice it to say that the following roles exist as great alternative careers in the medical field: dentist, nurse, nurse practitioner, physician's assistant, pharmacist, physical therapist, occupational therapist, clinical psychologist, nutritionist, audiologist, speech therapist, and more. All these roles involve direct patient interaction and are important components of medical care for many patients. Given that they all differ in the type of care administered and the length/cost of training, it is worthwhile to consider whether one of these healthcare professions may be a good fit for your goals. Feel free to skip forward to Chapter 7 for an in-depth discussion of several of these career paths.

8. Consider sacrifices you are (or are not) willing to make.

The last step I would recommend completing is related to and intertwined with many of those that came before; yet it is important to consider this independently, to ensure that you are ready to make the sacrifices necessary to become a physician and practice successfully.

Time

First and foremost, are you willing to put in the necessary time to complete medical education and training? In order to become a physician, after undergrad you must spend a minimum of seven years (if pursuing a residency such as family medicine, internal medicine, or pediatrics) to a maximum of twelve years (if pursuing a subspecialized fellowship like interventional cardiology or a longer residency such as neurosurgery). These are years during which you must be ready to work hard for long hours in a challenging environment. On one hand, it will require sacrificing time with loved ones and will likely mean missing some major life moments, as we have discussed. On the other hand, it will be an exciting and rewarding time of rapid learning and personal growth. At the end of the day, it is part of the process that cannot be avoided, and it is up to you to determine whether you are willing to make that commitment.

Money

The second consideration is money. We have so far covered the financial priorities and goals well-suited to a career in medicine. In Chapter 12, we will more deeply discuss the financial ramifications of medical education and training, including debt and opportunity cost. As a physician, you will certainly be well-compensated eventually; but there is no doubt that you will have to wait. Most will need to live somewhat frugally for the first several years until they reach an attending physician salary and are afforded more financial freedom. Again, this is an unpleasant but real challenge that can rarely be avoided on the path to becoming a physician. It pays to be aware and mentally prepared for this experience from the outset.

Make sure you are ready for these commitments—and sacrifices—before you choose a career in medicine. If prepared for them, and bolstered by the knowledge that medicine is a great fit for many of the reasons we previously discussed, you will not falter when you reach these hurdles. You will clear them steadily, one by one, and continue racing toward a successful career in medicine.

9. **Once you have decided, set your mind and your heart to the pursuit of medicine. You will not be stopped.**

This last step is self-explanatory. If you have done the necessary soul-searching and self-evaluation to determine that a career as a physician is the right choice for you, then dedicate yourself fully to that pursuit. Know that no matter how challenging the process is, you will ultimately reach your goal. Run the race with your eyes set on the finish line but also enjoy the process. Because at the end of the day, it is a marathon not a sprint. There is beauty in the process, the learning and growth that occur along the way. If after all these steps, you know that medicine is right for you, nothing will stand in your way.

Chapter 6: Types of Physician Degrees

Now that you have tackled whether medicine is the right career choice, the next decision awaits you: which medical degree to pursue.

Some may not even know that there are different degree options that lead to a career as a physician; but different paths do exist, with subtle but meaningful differences. It is therefore instructive to be aware of each of them. Let's discuss the major degree options that one can choose in order to reach the hallowed physician status: MD, DO, MD-PhD, MD-MBA, MD-MPH, MD-MS, and BS-MD (or BS-DO).

MD (Medical Doctor)

The MD degree is of course a primary subject of this book, so we won't delve into great detail here. But is a reasonable to touch on a few concepts which provide an overview and some historical context of this degree in the landscape of American medical education.

The MD degree is based on education of what is called *allopathic medicine,* or the treatment of medical disease with medications, surgery, radiation, and conventional medical therapies. It is what many describe colloquially as western medicine or modern medicine, (as opposed to eastern or naturopathic medicine). Currently there are 155 allopathic medical schools in the US, all of which confer the MD degree to graduates. Meanwhile, there are thirty-eight osteopathic medical schools in the US which confer the DO degree (more on this in a moment). There are also dozens of allopathic medical schools located in the Caribbean, a handful of which are more highly reputed. We will touch more on these in Chapter 9; but the primary focus of this book is US allopathic medical schools (MD programs) as well as US osteopathic medical schools (DO degree), as the experiences of students, residents and physicians from both of these pathways are quite similar.

MD programs last four years, typically comprised of two years of classroom, lab, and practical learning followed by two years of clinical rotations in clinics/hospitals. Graduates of MD programs can move onto residency and fellowship training in any specialty without restrictions. MD programs do vary in terms of acceptance rates, but all are quite competitive to gain acceptance to and are the most competitive in the spectrum of US medical degrees.

In the chapters that follow, we will closely examine the MD degree and the subsequent steps of a physician career thereafter. The information presented correlates most closely to the MD pathway (my experience and most common for physicians in the US) but is representative of the DO experience as well. Let's now examine osteopathic medicine and further discuss the similarities and differences between the MD and DO degree.

DO (Doctor of Osteopathic Medicine)

The DO degree is the slightly lesser-known partner of the MD degree, both of which culminate in a career as a practicing physician. A graduate with a DO degree is a full-fledged physician with all the same qualifications to practice medicine and care for patients as an MD. This is the first and most important fact to be aware of, which may be news to some. But what is osteopathy then, and how do the degrees differ?

Osteopathic medicine came into being in the late nineteenth century[1] and is a close relative of allopathic medicine, the traditional type of medicine taught in MD programs. As mentioned prior, in allopathic medicine, practitioners treat disease with medications, surgery, radiation, and other interventions. Osteopathic medicine also employs these approaches but adds alternative components such as osteopathic manipulation and a focus on preventative medicine (medical care geared toward preventing rather than treating medical disease)[1]. Osteopathic medicine has grown alongside allopathic medicine and they coexist today, though allopathic medicine is more widely taught and practiced. As of 2022, there are thirty-eight accredited DO schools in the US, comprising about twenty-five percent of currently enrolled US medical students[2].

MD and DO programs share many similarities as they are both four-year medical degrees, covering much of the same material and curriculum in the first two years followed by clinical rotations in years three and four. Yet they do differ fundamentally in a few ways.

First is the competitiveness of acceptance. DO programs have lower average Medical College Admissions Test (MCAT) scores and grade point average (GPA) than MD programs and are therefore considered somewhat less competitive to gain acceptance to. In 2018-2019, the average GPA and MCAT score for students accepted to DO schools were 3.54 and 503.8 respectively, compared to 3.72 and 511.2 for MD schools[3]. However, DO schools are still quite competitive, and ultimately provide good education and an excellent pathway to medical practice.

The second difference is educational focus. Much of the material covered in DO and MD schools is the same, with the exception of osteopathic manipulative medicine (OMM). Perhaps the most unique aspect of DO schools, OMM is the practice of manual manipulation of muscles, bone, and joints as a means of medical therapy. DO schools teach modern allopathic medicine in the same way that MD schools do, but integrate the alternative educational aspects of OMM to create a slightly different therapeutic skillset. Consequently, DO students are required to take a different set of board exams than MD students called COMLEX (Comprehensive Osteopathic Medical Licensing Examination). Most DO students opt to take both COMLEX and the US Medical Licensing Exam (USMLE), as it is beneficial to have USMLE exam scores to match into some residencies, particularly in competitive specialties. Of note, DOs and MDs are eligible to attend the same residency programs and there is technically no distinction made between them once they have graduated from medical school and begun residency training.

One fundamental point to be aware of is that attending DO vs. MD school can potentially change your ability to match into certain specialties and thus your possible career options. As mentioned, DOs can practice medicine in all the same ways that MDs can, without restriction. They even practice alongside

MDs in many clinics and hospitals. I have personally worked with several outstanding DOs. Thus, it is a misconception that their scope of practice differs from that of MDs. With that said, attending an osteopathic medical school does affect your chances of matching into residency in certain subspecialties. More than one third of DO students go on to practice primary care[1] (family medicine, internal medicine, and pediatrics). DO students can also apply to residencies in other specialties, but it is significantly harder to match into competitive residency programs and specialties as a DO than as a MD. For example, many top internal medicine programs historically do not accept DO applicants. Similarly, competitive specialties such as orthopedic surgery, head and neck surgery, plastic surgery, and dermatology (to name a few) may be exceedingly difficult to match into from an osteopathic medical school. One should be aware of this fact when applying to schools. If you know that you are targeting one of these specialties or programs, perhaps a DO degree is not the right fit for you. For others, it may be an ideal fit for their career goals and interests.

MD-PhD

The MD-PhD is perhaps a better-known alternative medical degree which premed students can choose to apply for. As its name implies, the degree is a combination of two doctorates, the medical doctor (MD) degree and the Doctor of Philosophy (PhD) degree. It is quite an undertaking and a significant accomplishment to earn an MD-PhD degree. In some ways, it is a herculean feat. Let's examine why.

The MD-PhD degree is typically eight to nine years total, consisting of four years of traditional medical school training and four to five years (perhaps longer if needed) to complete the PhD. Students begin medical school and complete the first two years of preclinical education along with their traditional

MD compatriots. After year two, MD-PhD students halt their medical training and begin graduate studies and lab work necessary to complete a PhD. This usually lasts around four to five years as mentioned. After completion of the PhD, MD-PhD students rejoins a new batch of med students to complete years three and four of medical school, consisting of clinical rotations (more on this in Chapter 9).

An important factor to be aware of when it comes to the MD-PhD degree is that the admissions process is highly competitive, even more competitive than that of traditional MD programs (as if it couldn't get any harder, right?). MD-PhD students are often the cream of the crop academically, with average GPA and MCAT scores even higher than MD students[4]. But after this added admissions hurdle, MD-PhD programs have the benefit of being completely funded in most cases. This means that most MD-PhD students have a full scholarship (and sometimes a stipend), saving tens of thousands of dollars on medical school tuition.

As anyone can see, this degree takes true dedication and is not for the faint of heart. It is nearly a decade-long process just to complete the education, after which residency would begin for those pursuing clinical practice. Typically, students who complete this degree have a deep interest in biomedical research, often basic science; but PhD pathways also exist in fields such as engineering, economics, epidemiology, or anthropology, to complement the medical degree. MD-PhD students will likely identify their passion early, and only strive for this degree if their passion is commensurate with the hard work and patience that the path requires. For others, I would advise caution when considering this degree. Be sure that you have a good reason to do so. Research can always be completed as a physician without a PhD; but if you do have a desire to pursue research very actively, to push the medical field forward through basic science research or to run your own lab, then this degree may be right for you. It can provide you with the education and skillset you need to do all the above and more.

Combined MD-Master's Degrees

A minority of students elect to pursue combined MD-Master's degrees, but for some with specific career goals this option may be a good fit.

The MD-MBA (Master of Business Administration) degree is growing in popularity, as the world of healthcare becomes increasingly intertwined with finance, business, and administration. This degree varies in format at different institutions but is generally five years total (traditional four years of medical school plus about one additional year for MBA degree). Students pursuing this degree may have an interest in the business and operations side of healthcare and may have their eyes set on hospital administration, consulting, or other non-clinical roles within medicine. Though it will require additional time and money, it may be a worthwhile investment for those with the appropriate career goals.

Meanwhile, the MD-MPH (Master of Public Health) degree is an opportunity for students interested in community and population health. This degree is also five years in duration, with one year of master's education in addition to the normal four years of medical school. The degree equips students with education regarding not only treatment of the individual patient, but management of patient populations as well as community-based interventions. Students graduating with this education may consider work in public health organizations, epidemiological research, or community-based health organizations, to name a few. Similarly, the MD-MPP (Master of Public Policy) degree provides additional education on analyzing and developing public policy, which can be a valuable skillset for advocacy work in the public sector, government, or nonprofit organizations. For students with an eye for big-picture, population-level interventions in addition to individual patient care, these degrees may be a worthwhile pursuit.

Finally, some students elect to pursue a MD-MS (Master of Science) degree. This pairs medical school with a master's degree, typically one year in duration and often completed in clinical research. This could be pursued by a medical trainee with an interest and eye for research who did not pursue a full PhD degree. Perhaps their passion for research was sparked after starting medical school, or perhaps they developed specific goals which a master's would sufficiently achieve without pursuing a full PhD. This additional training can bolster skills in research, statistics, and data analysis, and perhaps help launch a career as a clinician-investigator (a physician who works both clinically with patients and as a researcher investigating scientific questions).

Ultimately, within the scope of the medical degree, there are subtle differences and nuanced paths which can provide additional skillsets via extra training. By no means should a student feel compelled to pursue these. In fact, the majority of physicians do not. But it is advantageous to be aware of these options early on, as identifying any specific interests will allow you to pursue the degree which is best fit to your career goals.

Combined Undergraduate/Physician Degrees (BS-MD, BS-DO)

The final (and perhaps most unique/uncommon) route to a career as a physician is via a combined undergraduate-medical degree. These programs allow applicants to be admitted to both an undergrad degree (typically a Bachelor of Science) and a medical degree (either MD or DO) at once with only one application. In other words, a graduating high school student can apply for a combined BS-MD program and be accepted to both at the same time (typically at a single university). Once accepted, the student would no longer have to apply to medical school later on, as they would be guaranteed admission as long as they perform well and continue appropriately along their educational path during undergrad. These programs are typically seven to eight years (three to four years of undergrad plus four years of medical school), with a select few being only six years (two years of undergrad plus four years of medical school).

Combined Bachelor's-MD and Bachelor's-DO programs are significantly less common than the traditional route of undergraduate studies followed later by medical school via the usual application process. With that said, there are several combined program options available. In 2022, the Association of American Medical Colleges (AAMC) listed forty-five options for BS-MD programs[5], and several BS-DO programs exist as well. These programs tend to have a very competitive application process, often with very low acceptance rates. There are certainly some benefits to this pathway which include the potential to save one to two years of education (in six- or seven-year programs) as well as removing the huge challenge of getting accepted to medical school separately. But some downsides should also be considered: once accepted, the student is committed to that program and city for several years and will not have the opportunity to apply to other medical schools. The programs can be quite rigorous, and they require a significant, multi-year commitment at an early age (typically age seventeen or eighteen, when finishing high school). For those who are absolutely certain that a career as a physician is right for them, and reach this conclusion early on, these programs may be a great option. But I would heed caution for those who still need time to explore their interests and understand their personal and professional goals. Locking into up to eight years of education and deciding on the path to medical school so early should only be done by those who are truly sure, hopefully those who have already done much of the self-reflection we have discussed in this book.

There are several degree options which premeds can complete to reach their goal of becoming a physician, each with their own benefits and nuances. It is useful to be aware of all these options when deciding on how to pursue this complex career. In the next chapter, we will discuss an even broader consideration: alternative professions within healthcare, for those who are not completely decided on life as a physician.

Chapter 7: Alternative Career Paths Within Healthcare

Some individuals may hold a firm resolve that if they pursue healthcare, a career as a physician is the only path for them. For others who may be less certain, it is very reasonable to consider other potential healthcare professions besides a career as a medical doctor. Through evaluation of the alternatives, one can find which option fits their individual goals and interests best. We will discuss other health professional roles here so that aspiring premed students have a full lay of the land. Let's consider each option and discuss the pros, cons, similarities, and differences among them.

Dentist (DDM)

Undergraduate degree required? Yes
Education after undergrad: Four years of dental school
Residency: Optional (typically one to three years if chosen)
Cost: Comparable to medical school, but higher cost per year on average[1]. Also, some dental residencies cost additional tuition rather than paying the resident a salary. Thus, cost and debt incurred can be greater than physician training[1].
Competitiveness: High (though lower than medical school)

Dentistry is a great career option for those interested in healthcare, with broad patient care opportunities and a strong financial outlook. There are key differences between a career as a physician and dentist, some obvious and others less so. First, the obvious: dentistry is a heavily procedure-oriented profession with less breadth/scope of opportunity than medical practice, as it pertains to a particular portion of the body. Many medical specialties, such as primary care or radiology, would have far fewer hands-on procedures than dentistry, whereas surgical and procedural medical specialties would be comparable.

Perhaps less obvious is the difference in practice models and delivery of care. Contrary to medicine, dentistry is performed primarily in private practice settings, either individual or small group. Most dentists start their own practice or buy a share in an existing practice, while some dentists do work for larger entities such as a hospital or medical system. As you have likely experienced in your own life, it is more common to go to the individual private practice dentist than to a private practice physician. Dentistry has not had the same degree of transition to large group practice that medicine has. Thus, owning and running your own business (private practice) is more common in dentistry than in medicine. This is neither better nor worse, simply different; but this is an important facet of dentistry that one should be aware of, as different individuals may be more or less interested in this model of career practice.

As mentioned above, dental school (and even dental residency) can be more expensive than medical school, but typically requires fewer years of postgraduate/residency training. A general dentist can practice without any residency training or can opt for one year of general dentistry residency. Oral and maxillofacial surgery (OMFS, a subspecialty of dental surgery) on the other hand requires long and rigorous training which consists of four to six years of residency. Graduating students can enter OMFS residency from either dental or medical school, and some students attend programs at which they earn both degrees (MD and DDM). Other subspecialties of dentistry also require residency training: endodontics (two to three years), periodontics (three years), prosthodontics (three years), orthodontics (two to three years), and pediatric dentistry (two years). There is a range of subspecialties within dentistry with varying lengths of residency training, providing many options for the graduating dental student. Dentist salaries are quite variable by geography and specialty, so it is difficult to generalize; but the national median dentist salary has been reported at $190,000 as of 2023[2], slightly below average physician salaries. The potential for profit in a private practice setting or in specialties like dental surgery is quite high though, and thus there is considerable financial upside to this career.

Pharmacist (PharmD)

Undergraduate degree required? Yes
Education after undergrad: Four years of pharmacy school
Residency: Optional (one to two years)
Cost: Comparable to medical school (four years of education)
Competitiveness: Medium-High (though lower than medical school)

Pharmacy school is another great fit for individuals with an intellectual interest in medicine and the human body. One of the potential draws of pharmacy school to interested premeds may be that much of the foundational physiology, pathophysiology, and pharmacology are the same as those learned in medical school. The pharmacist then develops more subspecialized knowledge about medicines and therapeutics; but there are many parallels between the learning process of pharmacy and medical education. One major difference between the two careers is that, in general, a physician will ultimately have much more hands-on patient interaction.

Pharmacists practice in varied settings, from local pharmacies such as those at CVS or Rite-Aid to outpatient clinics to hospitals. In each setting, they utilize different skillsets and knowledge. Pharmacy school graduates can practice in local pharmacies and some other settings without any residency training. Those who do wish to pursue further specialty training can complete residencies of one to two years in varying subspecialties which mirror those of medicine. This allows them to practice in a variety of clinical settings, such as emergency medicine, critical care, or ambulatory (outpatient) care. The variety of practice settings in pharmacy again makes it difficult to characterize their average pay, but the national median salary is around $149,00 based on data published in 2023[3]. With shorter training (no required residency) and a solid eventual salary, pharmacy may be a good option for those with a particular interest in pharmacology but less desire for patient care.

Optometrist (OD)

Undergraduate degree required? Yes
Education after undergrad: Four years of optometry school
Residency: Optional (one year)

Cost: Comparable to medical school (four years of education), but slightly lower per year cost on average[4]
Competitiveness: Medium

Optometry is a unique career option within the healthcare field, holding some of the same benefits and distinctions as dentistry. Much like a dentist, an optometrist can practice independently at the top of their line of work, without oversight from a physician or other medical professional. Furthermore, within optometry lies a significant opportunity for private practice, a chance to run your own business and be your own boss. Along with this opportunity come challenges, but there are certainly positive aspects to the private practice model as previously discussed. Optometrists can also join a group practice or clinic rather than start their own practice, providing multiple potential settings in which to work. Because of the opportunity to run their own practice/business, there may be significant variability in optometrist salaries. National data indicates that the median salary for optometrists in 2022 was approximated $133,000[5].

Clinically, optometrists have a significant amount of direct patient care, working daily with patients to treat various eye conditions. An important distinction to be aware of, which may not be immediately obvious to most, is the functional difference between optometry and ophthalmology. These are two completely separate fields, with different educational and training paths, but both treat ailments of the eye. An ophthalmologist is an MD who has attended four years of medical school and subsequently completed four years of residency training (three of them in ophthalmology). Ophthalmologists use medications and perform surgeries to treat diseases of the eye, from cataracts to infections to trauma and more. Optometrists, on the other hand, are not MD's but hold the degree of OD. They have completed four years of optometry school and have the option to complete an additional one year of residency training. Optometrists focus primarily on treatment of refractive errors of the eye such as nearsightedness, farsightedness, and astigmatism with the use of eyeglasses and contact lenses. They do not perform surgeries. Though optometrists do treat some other maladies of the eye, they have a more limited/focused scope of practice than an ophthalmologist. These two fields differ greatly in both training and practice, but each plays an important role in the care of eye disorders.

Physician Assistant (PA)

Undergraduate degree required? Yes
Education after undergrad: Two to three years of PA school, length depending on the program
Residency: Optional (one to two years)
Cost: Lower than medical school (fewer years of education)
Competitiveness: Medium

A career as a Physician Assistant (PA) is one of the closest matches to that of a physician, as the name implies. PAs works closely alongside physicians and provide direct patient care in both inpatient and outpatient settings. In some ways, a PA functions like a resident in that they see patients, write orders and notes, and provide medical care, but do so under the tutelage and guidance of a supervising physician. The path to becoming a PA is certainly much shorter and cheaper than physician training, with only two to three years of PA school and no residency required thereafter. PA residencies are available in subspecialties and generally last one to two years but are not required for clinical practice. The shorter duration of training may be appealing to an individual who knows they want to care for patients the way a physician does, but without enduring the minimum of seven (up to a maximum of twelve) years of training after undergrad which are required to become an attending physician.

While demanding less training and lower cost, bear in mind that the pay for a PA is significantly lower than that of a physician (as would be expected). PA salaries vary by state and specialty with average salaries ranging from about $78,000 per year in North Carolina to about $125,00 per year in New York, according to data published in 2023[6]. This is certainly a good wage and can be a comfortable living. It is interesting to note that, on average, this is a considerably higher starting salary than most resident physician positions across the country. A benefit of a career as a PA is that there is opportunity to move laterally across specialties. In other words, a PA is not bound to one specialty as a physician is (unless the physician goes back to repeat residency or a different fellowship, which is a huge undertaking). For example, a PA can start working in inpatient cardiology and later move to outpatient oncology. There is significant professional flexibility in this career, which may be a positive aspect for those interested. One practical consideration about a career as a PA is reduced autonomy, which would be expected given much shorter training. Though PAs are capable and important medical providers, they will not have the same level of autonomous practice and decision-making as a physician. If independent practice is important to you, perhaps the additional time required to become a physician is worth it. If not, a career as a PA may be a great fit.

Nurse Practitioner (MSN or DNP)

Undergraduate degree required? Yes

Education after undergrad: Two to four years, length depending on the degree/program. Typically, two to three years for MSN degree (Master of Science in Nursing) and

three to four years for DNP degree (Doctor of Nursing Practice)[7].
Residency: Optional
Cost: Comparable to medical school, though may be lower given possibility of only three years of education
Competitiveness: Medium

Another great option for those who want to pursue patient care which is similar to that of a physician is becoming a nurse practitioner (NP). Though there are significant educational/training differences between NP and physician degrees, NPs are able to work alongside physicians providing patient care; depending on the geographic location and clinical situation, they can even practice independently. NPs work in both inpatient and outpatient settings. They typically work alongside a supervising physician, but twenty-two states currently allow NPs to work independently of physicians[8]. Therefore, NPs have greater opportunity for autonomy than PAs. A quick word on this though: remember that if you have a specific goal which requires advanced practice, you may only be able to achieve that goal through physician training. For example, though NPs and PAs can work as surgical assistants and care for pre- and post-operative patients, they will not be able to independently operate as a surgeon does. Thus, this career provides opportunity for autonomy but with logical and necessary limitations. Keep this in mind when considering your personal goals. Much like PAs, NPs have significant professional flexibility in that they can change specialties during their career. Though there is always a learning curve when moving to a new field, NPs do not have to go back to repeat school or a residency/fellowship in order to change to a new specialty. This is a significant benefit of the shorter training/reduced autonomy of the NP and PA degrees. As with PAs, the average salary for NPs is certainly lower than that of physicians but generally sits well above the six-figure mark (approximately $123,000 in 2021)[9]. Thus, it can be a lucrative career that offers patient care and opportunity for autonomy, with shorter education/training.

Registered Nurse (ADN, BSN, or MSN)

Undergraduate degree required? Maybe
Education: Varies depending on degree. Associate's Degree in Nursing (ADN) can be done instead of a Bachelor's (meaning you do not need to go to undergrad) and typically lasts two years. Bachelor's of Science in Nursing (BSN) can be completed during undergrad (four years) or post-undergrad (typically one to two additional years). Master's of Science in Nursing (MSN) is two additional years after undergrad.
Residency: None
Cost: Lower than medical school (fewer years of education)
Competitiveness: Low-Medium (depending on the type of degree and competitiveness of program)

Nurses are, without a doubt, the backbone of the healthcare system. They play a crucial and indispensable role and often do not get enough recognition for their contributions. That is changing to a degree based on greater societal awareness of the healthcare system and thus the importance of nurses, particularly during the COVID-19 pandemic. But let me take a strong and clear stance here: nursing is a highly respectable and noble profession. It is an outstanding way to help patients and contribute to the healthcare field.

The path to becoming a nurse varies based on which route is taken. Understanding the world of nursing can be difficult, as there are multiple healthcare professional roles which are similar to, but not the same as, the registered nurse. First let us understand the basic nomenclature.

Registered Nurse (RN) is the designation for a fully functioning nurse who works with patients in conjunction with a physician, with no additional nursing oversight. This is what people typically envision when talking about nursing practice.

Licensed vocational nurse (LVN) or licensed practical nurse (LPN) are designations for individuals who work with patients under the supervision of a physician but often also supervised by an RN. LVNs/LPNs have somewhat shorter training (typically one year total) and consequently less scope of practice, less independence, and lower average pay than RNs.

Certified nursing assistant (CNA) is a nursing professional who assists RNs and LVNs with a number of nursing tasks including taking vital signs, bathing/cleaning patients, providing medications, and more.

For the purposes of this text, I will focus on the RN which is the highest education/training designation for a bedside nurse. One can become an RN by way of an ADN, BSN, or MSN degree. Average annual salaries for RNs range from about $58,000 to $106,000[10] depending on the state of employment. Nurses are paid hourly, so the salary will depend on the typical RN workweek of thirty-six to forty hours. Of note, there are opportunities for considerably higher pay when working in areas with nursing shortages, such as travel nursing or work in underserved areas. RNs, particularly in the inpatient setting, have perhaps the greatest opportunity for direct patient contact of any healthcare professional; nurses are the ones at the bedside providing the majority of the day-to-day and hour-to-hour patient care. Consequently, nurses have a job which is both challenging and rewarding. For those interested in an alternative to becoming a physician which provides the opportunity to truly touch the lives of patients, nursing is a great option that warrants consideration.

Physical Therapist (DPT)

Undergraduate degree required? Yes
Education after undergrad: Three years of physical therapy school
Residency: None
Cost: Lower than medical school (fewer years of education)
Competitiveness: Medium

Physical therapy offers a unique and impactful way to provide patient care. It is a field that offers a variety of practice settings including both inpatient and outpatient care. In the inpatient setting, physical therapists focus mostly on restoring mobility and function for patients who are debilitated from injury, illness, deconditioning from the hospitalization, or all the above. In the outpatient setting, physical therapists work to improve strength/function for muscles and joints, treating a multitude of musculoskeletal injuries. Outpatient therapists sometimes have the opportunity to work with athletes rehabilitating from injury or surgery, which can be an exciting part of the job. With expertise in joint injuries and overlap with sports medicine, physical therapy can be an intriguing option for those who are interested in the intersection of medicine and athletics.

Training to become a physical therapist requires three years of graduate school with both classroom and clinical training. Average annual salaries range from approximately $76,000 to $100,000 based on state of employment[11]. One aspect to note about physical therapy is that it focuses on non-pharmacologic treatments (i.e. therapies and exercises rather than medications), which may be a downside if you have a particular interest in pharmacology or physiology. On the other hand, for those who have greater interest in anatomy and kinesiology, this profession may be a great fit.

Clinical Psychologist (Psy.D or PhD)

Undergraduate degree required? Yes
Education after undergrad: Variable depending on institution and exact degree. Requires a doctorate in Psychology (four to seven years). Some doctorate programs also require a Master's in Psychology for acceptance (two additional years).
Residency: No formal residency, but doctorate degree contains a clinical internship. Some states require additional clinical hours (up to one to two years) after education to perform independent clinical practice.
Cost: Variable, but lower cost per year than medical school. PhD degrees often come with a significant amount of funding which reduces cost for the student. Fewer funding opportunities exist for the Psy.D degree.
Competitiveness: Medium

A career as a clinical psychologist is another intriguing option for individuals looking for a profession rich in patient care. Clinical psychology is actually very diverse in terms of educational paths and career possibilities. We will not touch on all these nuances; rather, I will focus on the path of the licensed clinical psychologist, which is the highest professional designation. Becoming a licensed clinical psychologist requires completion of an undergraduate degree (typically a psychology major is encouraged) followed by a doctorate in Psychology. The doctorate degree can either be a PhD or a Psy.D, either of which typically takes about four to seven years to complete. The PhD degree is geared more towards education and research, while the Psy.D focuses on clinical practice. Some psychology doctorate programs also require a master's degree for acceptance (another two years typically)[12].

Similar to the distinction between optometry and ophthalmology, it is important to note the difference between a clinical psychologist and a psychiatrist. A psychiatrist is a physician who completed medical school and then residency in psychiatry. They diagnose and treat patients with a variety of mental illness, using medications as well as counseling and therapeutic techniques. Meanwhile, a clinical psychologist can see patients and manage illnesses such as anxiety and depression through counseling, psychotherapy, and other means; but in most cases, clinical psychologists cannot prescribe medications as a psychiatrist (MD) does. Thus, a clinical psychologist's scope of practice lies more in counseling and techniques such as cognitive behavioral therapy/other psychotherapies. Clinical psychologists can also pursue other professional roles such as educational counseling, forensic psychology, or psychology services in industry/business.

Clinical psychology is a unique and diverse professional field. It does require a long road of training, comparable though on average shorter than physician training. Salaries vary based upon the professional setting in which the psychologist practices but are lower on average than physician salaries, with the national average salary around $102,000 per year in 2022[13]. This dynamic field may be a good consideration for anyone with significant interest in neuroscience, psychology, and patient care.

As we have seen through this discussion, there are a multitude of professional options within the healthcare field, each with pros, cons, and varying levels of investment/ultimate reward. The goal of this chapter was to equip readers with knowledge of the major professional options that exist within healthcare. Due to the breadth of the medical field, we are unable to cover every healthcare job but touched on the key ones that could be viable alternatives for premed students. Other pathways which we did not discuss include audiology, speech pathology, respiratory therapy, clinical nutrition, and more. These roles are typically considered support services meant to complement the care of the primary medical provider, but they are nonetheless integral components of the healthcare system which provide important services to patients.

I strongly encourage all students to pursue whatever profession is the best fit for their interests, personal priorities, and career goals. These personal priorities are what matter most. Whether you chose to become a physician, another healthcare provider, or any other professional, remember two things along the way: hard work, dedication, and perseverance will ultimately be rewarded; and attention to your own goals and values, both personal and professional, will provide the best foundation for sustainable happiness.

Part III: Pursuit

Chapter 8: What is Premed Really Like?

We have covered a great deal so far, primarily related to the mental preparatory work that should be done before choosing to pursue a career as a physician. Now we will move on to an exciting portion of our discussion: what the path of a physician actually looks and feels like. We will consider in detail the experience of the journey through a medical career: the premed years, medical school, residency training, and physician practice. In doing so, premeds will develop a much more thorough understanding of a potential future in this profession. For others not pursuing a medical career, these descriptions may facilitate a better understanding of what a friend, loved one, or even your own doctor experienced on the road to where they are today.

College Year One

For some, the premedical experience starts as early as high school with volunteering or perhaps even a research job (yes, I have seen some high school students working in research labs!). These individuals start the process of exploring medicine early to increase their exposure. Kudos to them; but for most, the process starts in earnest with undergraduate studies. This is where we will begin our discussion.

Year one of undergrad, which kicks off the bulk of the premed experience, is characterized mostly by the adjustment to college life: to no longer having a parent to cook meals or do laundry; to living with your friends and being able to spend your time however you please; to figuring out how to navigate the rigors of college academics while enjoying social life on campus. Newfound opportunity and responsibility are the underlying themes of the first year of college for any eager freshman stepping on campus.

Specific to the experience of the premed, the name of the game is academic performance. In the first year, among the many fun experiences of college, you will be focused on studying hard and scoring well enough on your exams to maintain a high GPA. This is really the most important goal in the beginning of undergrad, as falling behind with a low GPA early on can be tough to recover from later. Maintaining your grades will be stressed by mentors and advisors for good reason. It is no secret that medical school acceptance is very challenging: in 2020 the average acceptance rate was about six percent for the 121 ranked MD medical schools, with the top schools' acceptance rates hovering around two percent[1]. In recent years, about forty percent of all MD medical school applicants achieve acceptance annually[2]. A high GPA is one of the most important factors in the application. Therefore, a premed will have to make sure that amidst the fun and games (of which there can be plenty), they achieve the grades needed to keep them in the running for medical school applications down the line.

Coursework during this first year will be rigorous. Although one can choose any major and still apply to med school—yes, anything from philosophy to computer science to human physiology—all premeds will need to complete the prerequisite classes for medical school applications. These include biology, physical chemistry, organic chemistry, physics, and calculus; prerequisite coursework will amount to about one year of each of these subjects. The classes are challenging and can be competitive, so they will require focus and discipline. They will also hopefully be fun and interesting, especially in the case of courses pertaining closely to medicine, such as human physiology.

College Year Two

Year two of college is an academic continuation of what was described above. It generally takes about two years to complete the premed prerequisites, so students will continue on the quest to master these subjects and capture a high GPA.

What is more unique about this year is that generally premed students begin seeking out the practical experience/exposure we have previously discussed—volunteer positions, shadowing, and research. When I advise/mentor students, I always recommend that they begin the process of searching for these positions by late first year so that they can be in full swing by year two. Second year if college is one of the most pivotal steps in the premed process, as gaining these experiences accomplishes two things: first, it helps advance the process of exploring medicine described in Chapter 5, providing the tangible exposure that students need to determine if life as a physician is a good fit; second, it achieves the volunteer and clinical experiences necessary to submit a competitive med school application when the student is ready.

Year two of college will be that exciting time of gaining the exposure needed to truly evaluate a career in medicine. It is prudent to seek a clinical role (either volunteer work, shadowing, or both) as well as a research role (basic science or clinical). Most students who will ultimately be successful in their med school applications will accomplish both sometime around the middle years of college.

Please note that while I delineate the year-by-year steps on the path to becoming a physician, the first two to three years of undergrad are the time when individuals should be exploring both medicine and themselves to determine if they truly want to become a physician. This will be an ongoing process. No student should ever be expected to know definitively on day one of college (or even later) whether they want to become a physician. Many who may think they know for sure will have a change of heart or circumstance, and this is absolutely okay. This self-discovery will be an evolving process. By going through it, one way or another, you will find the path that is best for you.

College Year Three

For most premed students, the focus during year three of college shifts to the MCAT (Medical College Admissions Test), which is the standardized exam for medical school acceptance. This exam is analogous to the SAT or ACT exams taken during high school for college applications. The MCAT allows medical schools to compare all applicants on a common, standardized measure. Rather than using only GPA, given that the grading and rigor of courses can vary between institutions, schools also use the MCAT as a benchmark of academic performance that applies more equally to students across all campuses. For this reason, the stakes for this exam are high. This is by far the single most important exam you will take prior to medical school, and it should be treated with commensurate respect. The MCAT score will be one of the largest components of your medical school application. Without an adequate one, acceptance to medical school will be a much taller task.

This is not meant to intimidate, but to accurately highlight the importance of this exam. The MCAT is difficult, but with hard work and preparation, you can certainly succeed. The exam is a multiple choice, computer-based test taken at standardized testing centers on dates offered throughout the year. It lasts seven and a half hours; this may be a staggering number to some who have not taken a test of this length before. Though this type of exam is grueling, as I can attest to from personal experience, do not fret about this number. Prior to the exam, you will be well-prepared by diligent studying and deliberate development of testing stamina. Similar to a marathon runner training with sequential increases in running length, the student should prepare with sequential increases in studying/test-taking duration. With the right training, you will carefully prepare for this exam duration and be ready to go when test day arrives.

The MCAT is composed of four sections which cover the following: biology and biochemistry; chemistry and physics; psychology and sociology; critical analysis and reasoning. The entire exam is multiple choice (there is no longer a written section as there used to be).

We cover this information here to give you an overview of the MCAT, but do not get bogged down by the details at this point. It is sufficient for now to know that the exam will require significant planning and preparation. Most premeds who plan to apply to medical school during or shortly after college will take the MCAT during their third year. You may notice that many of the prerequisite courses I described in years one and two of undergrad are represented on the MCAT; thus, it makes sense for most students to take the MCAT shortly after completing the bulk of these courses. With that said, these courses alone are not adequate preparation for the MCAT. Students will need to put in dozens (maybe hundreds) of hours of independent study using books and often formal courses. I will leave the determination of how to study for the MCAT to the individual student, as this decision depends on your own study habits and preferences. There is a plethora of resources available for MCAT preparation. I suggest that when the time comes, you consider at least some of them.

Somewhere around year three of college is the right time to take the MCAT, though this is not set in stone by any means. Some students may even take the exam during the summer after year two (like myself) or later (in year four perhaps). If planning to take a gap year (or two) after college before applying to medical school, premeds have the flexibility to take this exam later. Any of these timing alterations are appropriate as long as they fit your personal goals and trajectory.

Year three of college will otherwise consist of finishing any remaining prerequisite courses, starting upper division college courses, and continuing research/clinical activities that were already ongoing. It will likely also contain some other extracurricular pursuits, as a complete medical school application really should consist of at least a handful of these activities. Hopefully, the year will also consist of some good, old-fashioned fun as you enjoy the great times of college life.

College Year Four

Year four of college will initially be a continuation of upper division coursework, research work, clinical experience, and any other volunteer or student organization involvement a student has chosen. It will also be a final year of good times spent with great friends. Cherish that—it is important, it is unique, and it is to be valued!

For many applicants (but not all), the final year of college will also be highlighted by applying to medical school. This will be an exciting and busy time, as the hard work of several prior years will culminate with medical school applications—and hopefully acceptance! Now keep in mind that the timing of medical school application is quite variable and, similar to the MCAT it, can be adjusted to the goals and preferences of the individual. Some choose to apply to medical school as early as possible (end of third year/beginning of fourth year of college) to avoid a gap year, but this is by no means necessary. A large portion of medical school applicants apply later; a 2019 survey by the American Medical Association (AMA) showed that forty-three percent of matriculating medical students took one to two gap years[3].

Though the med school application typically occurs during college or within the first one to two years after college, it can really be done at any time so long as the applicant has the appropriate experience and qualifications. According to the AMA, in 2019 the average age of matriculating medical students was twenty-four[4]. The AAMC similarly reported that in 2018, the median age of matriculating medical students was twenty-four, but ages ranged from twenty-one at the first percentile to forty at the ninety-ninth percentile[5]. These data demonstrate that a student can choose to apply to medical school whenever the time is right for them, based on their pre-existing experiences and current career goals. There is no harm in taking one or multiple gap years to either bolster an application or pursue other interests. In many cases, this may even strengthen the application through diverse life experiences.

With that said, a large portion of premeds will choose to apply to medical school during fourth year of college. We will not belabor all the details of the medical school application here as many other resources exist; but know that applications will consist of essentially seven major components, listed here in relative order of importance:

1. Undergraduate GPA
2. MCAT score
3. Clinical experience
4. Research experience
5. Personal statement
6. Letters of recommendation
7. Community service, alternative work experience, extracurricular activities, etc.

Each of these components will have been developed over the preceding years of undergraduate study. Upon reaching year four, students will essentially need to put it all together into a neat and effective package, a sales-pitch representing why you are a suitable candidate to join the medical profession.

Along these lines, the main tasks for year four of college will be to secure letters of recommendations (typically four to five from a combination of professors, research mentors, and clinical mentors), write a personal statement, and complete the primary medical school application itself (more on the secondary application soon). The primary application is a standardized application submitted to all medical schools, though there are separate applications for MD and DO programs. You must choose a list of schools to apply to and compose descriptions of all prior experiences in addition to your personal statement. This process generally takes one to two months, requiring careful work and ideally some deliberation with experienced mentors. Once complete, a student will submit the primary application to their schools of choice.

But wait...there's more! As if the first step was not enough, the applicant will then move onto the secondary application. Secondaries are a subsequent component of each application which is specific to the individual school. Many (but not all) schools will send a secondary to every applicant; some schools will screen applicants initially and only send secondaries to certain students. Secondary applications will consist mostly of additional essays (ironically, becoming a physician will require a lot of writing, at least up front). These essays will ask the applicant to answer prompts such as why they chose medicine, why they are a good fit for that program, and other questions regarding the individual's past experiences. The applicant will submit a separate secondary to each school which has requested one if they wish to proceed with that application.

Ah, now we're done, right? Almost, but not quite! The final step in the application process will be interviews. Though on the surface they may be anxiety-provoking, interviews are typically one of the most enjoyable parts of the medical school application process. Students historically got to travel to each medical school that offered them an interview (assuming there was not a pandemic in full swing requiring virtual interviews). They would visit each campus and meet the faculty and students in person. Though a considerable financial investment, this was a great opportunity to explore new parts of the country and get to know the nuances of potential programs. As a result of the COVID-19 pandemic, much of the traditional in-person interview process has been transitioned to virtual interviews. Some schools do still offer in-person options (or occasionally encourage it), but the majority rely primarily on virtual interviews currently. It is unclear whether this change will become permanent as a result of the pandemic. In my opinion, it is beneficial for applicants to get to visit different cities and campuses to decide which region and program is best for them. With that said, virtual interviews are considerably less expensive, and students will still get a feel for the program by meeting faculty and going through the orientation and information provided by the medical school.

The medical school application itself will cost several hundred to a few thousand dollars most likely, depending on the number of schools the student applies to and the number of interviews they attend in-person. This may sound daunting, and it is certainly not trivial; but ultimately it is a small portion of the total expense of medical training and is a necessary part of the process. Of note, there is a fee assistance program through the AAMC which provides financial aid for things such as the MCAT and med school applications (to MD programs) for those who qualify.

Now comes the final step: acceptance! Students will typically begin receiving acceptance letters as soon as the fall of fourth year (for those who submitted applications the summer before their fourth year, the earliest possible time). Letters will continue to arrive through the spring of fourth year (or the spring following the initial submission of the primary application). This will be a sweet and satisfying culmination of years of hard work and perseverance. Be sure to enjoy it, as it is well-deserved!

One important point to note here is that some applicants will decide later, after completing their initial college years, that they want to pursue a career as a physician. If the applicant did not complete the necessary prerequisite courses during undergrad (for example, if they were a humanities major and not a premed), they can pursue what is called a post-baccalaureate program. These are programs which are started after completing college, meaning the individual will need to go back to school. These programs are designed to specifically cover the course work needed to prepare for and apply to medical school. It is technically never too late to pursue a career as a physician, and there are many avenues to achieve acceptance!

Chapter 9: What is Medical School Really Like?

Success! If you've reached this stage of medical training, major congratulations are in order. It is no easy task to be accepted to medical school; it takes a tremendous amount of hard work, discipline, and patience, and you deserve to be recognized for that effort.

But make no mistake—the hard work does not stop here. There is certainly a myth out there that "getting into medical school is the hard part, and what follows is easier." Unfortunately, it is my responsibility to debunk that notion now. Medical school acceptance is certainly very difficult, but the road does not get easier going forward. Medical education and training are arduous throughout, as they must create well-trained and battle-tested physicians, capable of bearing the responsibility of caring for human lives.

With that said, getting accepted to medical school is perhaps the most important hurdle because it is the step at which the most people falter. With the overall acceptance rate for MD medical schools hovering at about forty annually, there is certainly a far higher attrition rate prior to medical school acceptance than after. (Unfortunately, there is some attrition after medical school acceptance as well, with the "drop-out" rate reported between fifteen and eighteen percent for four-year allopathic medical schools[1].) If you have made it this far, you have plenty of hard work to go, but you have secured your place in the cohort of medical professionals. You have achieved what I consider the "activation energy" of medical training. Now that this threshold level has been achieved, the subsequent "reaction" can proceed: beginning your medical education and continuing to succeed along the road to becoming a physician.

So, what is medical school really like? We will break down each year of med school into its key components to demystify the process of medical education. For many (including myself), med school was a well-known entity with equally poorly understood components. I knew that I was starting four years of intense studies and training; but honestly, I did not know much about what that experience would entail. It is your right to know what you or your loved ones are signing up for. It is time to get informed!

Before delving into the details of each year individually, it helps to have an initial overview of years one through four and their roles/functions. In essence, medical school is broken down as follows, with perhaps some minor variations at certain schools:

Years one and two are primarily classroom learning, a bit like undergrad "on steroids." This time will be spent learning the bread-and-butter medical knowledge needed for clinical practice. Most schools will have a small amount of clinical work in years one and two as well. This is an adjunct to the main classroom learning and is meant to kickstart the development of basic clinical skills. Typically, at the end of year two (though this may be somewhat variable by school), students will take Step 1 of the USMLE, a standardized exam for all medical students. The USMLE is a three-step exam meant to comprehensively assess the knowledge gained in medical school. Historically, Step 1 was the most important of the three exams, and the single most important exam of one's medical career (yes, even more so than the MCAT). Step 1 was a huge factor in residency applications and a large determinant of an applicant's future ability to match into a specialty; without an adequate score, certain specialty choices would not be attainable. But as of 2022, Step 1 of the USMLE became a pass/fail exam and is no longer numerically scored. Thus, it is now a lower stakes exam, though passing is still very important of course as it is necessary to move to the next step of medical training. With that said, this change undoubtedly places more weight and emphasis on the numerical score received on Step 2 of the USMLE, a two-part exam taken after third year of medical school. Step 2 has in a way become the new Step 1, at least in terms of the impact it has on residency applications. More detail on both exams come later in this chapter.

One other important point to note is that the USMLE exams are required for MD students. DO students are required to take a different three-part exam called COMLEX (Comprehensive Osteopathic Medical Licensing Examination). Many DO students end up taking both exams if hoping to apply to more competitive residencies which typically match MDs and may necessitate the USMLE.

Years three and four of medical school will switch gears almost completely. Students will leave the classroom and work full-time in hospitals and clinics. They will often work schedules similar to residents, at times approaching or exceeding eighty hours a week (though typically the medical student schedule is somewhat less rigorous than that of residents). The key to be aware of is that during these two years, medical students will *work* rather than simply *study*. It is a much different learning experience, both exciting and taxing in new ways. The learning never stops though. In fact, it likely increases during this time. Unfortunately, the tests continue as well, with major exams at the end of each clinical rotation.

During the third year of medical school, students rotate through all the major medical and surgical specialties to complete their general medical training. This broad experience allows students to lay the foundation of their medical skills and gain the exposure needed to choose their specialty for residency. During year four, students will take Step 2 of their medical boards. As mentioned, this exam historically has had two parts completed on different days: Step 2 Clinical Knowledge (CK) is a multiple-choice exam much like Step 1, while Step 2 Clinical Skills (CS) is a practical exam consisting of observed encounters with simulated patients (actors). Fourth year also consists of time for students to complete additional rotations in selected specialties (usually their planned residency specialty) along with some elective rotations.

Finally, students will apply to residency during fourth year and match into the specialty of their choosing at one particular program (more on this process later). And that'll be the end of it...until residency starts, of course, and the fun begins all over again!

Different Types of Medical Education: MD, DO, and Caribbean Medical Schools

Before understanding the process of medical school education, it is important to recognize that there are different types of medical schools with some key differences. As previously discussed in Chapter 6, there are two different types of medical schools within the US: ones that offer the Medical Doctor (MD) degree and ones that offer the Doctor of Osteopathy (DO) degree. It is important to remember that though two types of medical education exist, both degrees allow the graduate to fully practice medicine/patient care and to attend any type of residency training program. Despite subtle differences in education, DO programs provide all the standard medical education, and graduates of these programs can practice alongside MDs in the same capacity.

Another option for some US premed students is to attend medical school in the Caribbean, or even abroad in other countries. Caribbean medical schools provide an MD degree upon graduation. Students typically spend two years in the Caribbean completing classroom learning on campus and then move to various US hospitals for their clinical rotations during years three and four. Caribbean medical schools (and some DO programs) do not necessarily have one system of affiliated hospitals, as MD medical schools typically do. Therefore, students in year three and four typically travel to multiple different hospitals and cities to complete their clinical rotations.

Both DO and Caribbean schools are less competitive to gain acceptance to than MD schools, and thus can be an option for some students. Caribbean medical schools tend to have a higher attrition rate, meaning a lower percentage of their students graduate compared to traditional US medical schools. Upon graduating from these schools, it can also be more difficult to match into competitive residency specialties, similar to the discussion in Chapter 6 regarding DO schools. But many students do succeed at Caribbean or international medical schools and return to the US to have excellent careers. Depending on the student and their prior experience/academic background, Caribbean or international medical schools may be good options. What I will describe in the pages that follow is the typical experience at most MD schools, which make up the majority of US medical schools. There will be many similarities and common themes, but bear in mind that there will also be some differences at DO, Caribbean, or international medical schools, which we will not cover individually in depth.

Let's now take a more detailed look at the experience during each year of medical school.

Medical School Year One

Year one of medical school is what most people envision when they think of the experience. It primarily consists of a rigorous curriculum of coursework in some key subjects: anatomy, the study of the structure of the human body; physiology, the study of the function of each organ system of the human body; pathophysiology, the study of diseases and disorders that affect the different organ systems; and pharmacology, the study of medicines and treatments of disease. The vast majority of first-year coursework will fall into one of these categories, which lay the foundation of knowledge required to become a practicing physician.

Most medical schools now employ a combination of traditional, lecture-based learning with a significant component of what is called problem-based learning (PBL). This alternative method of education puts students in small groups (typically eight to ten people) with an instructor to review cases or clinical problems which simulate real medical practice. The cases illustrate key learning points which mirror the subjects being covered in parallel during the traditional course lectures. PBL introduces students to the process of applying medical knowledge to clinical situations through critical thinking and reasoning. Its goal is to build upon knowledge gained in lectures to create clinical reasoning applicable to real medical practice.

As is common knowledge to most, medical students will also go through a series of practical, hands-on classes. You have probably heard of anatomy lab. This is where students will dissect human cadavers to understand the intricacies of human anatomy, which is the scaffold over which all subsequent medical learning will be laid. This is a truly unforgettable and invaluable learning experience for every medical student. (Special thanks and recognition are necessary here to the generous souls who donated their bodies to medical science, helping train the next generation of physicians.) Most schools have similar practical courses for histology/pathology (the microscopic evaluation of tissue, which can be informative for diagnosis of many diseases) as well as microbiology (the study of infectious agents such as bacteria, viruses, and parasites).

Finally, students will complete a curriculum designed to teach the hard skills of clinical practice, including physical exam skills, the art of speaking with patients and obtaining a medical history, dealing with challenging patient situations, and more. This learning is geared toward the actual practice of medicine, helping students gain the tools necessary to assess and eventually treat patients in the real world. This curriculum typically employs periodic standardized patient encounters, during which students interact with actors playing the role of patients, in order to apply the skills they have learned to realistic clinical scenarios.

These components will make up the bulk of education in the first year of medical school, creating a rigorous schedule and an unprecedented amount of information to be learned. It is truly a new experience, with significantly greater pace and volume of learning than in undergrad. There will certainly be growing pains; most students need to adjust and refine their study skills to succeed. But once you find your rhythm, the first year of medical school is fascinating. It allows you to expand your knowledge by leaps and bounds, satisfying many of the intellectual curiosities which drove you to pursue medicine in the first place.

Medical School Year Two

Year two of medical school is punctuated most significantly by the USMLE Step 1 exam. Though it does not occur until late in the academic year, students will typically prepare for the Step 1 throughout the year. Meanwhile, coursework and learning continue in year two much as they did in year one. Year two typically contains a greater focus on pathophysiology and pharmacology, as students draw upon the foundation from year one to build knowledge of disease processes and their treatments. Throughout the year students will slowly ramp up their studying for the Step 1 exam, which typically occurs in the last one to two months of second year before transitioning to full-time clinical work in year three.

Step 1 of the USMLE is a one day, eight-hour exam consisting of a maximum of 280 questions. It is divided into seven testing blocks with a maximum of forty questions each[2]. All questions are multiple-choice and the majority are based on clinical scenarios. The exam covers essentially all the material from years one and two of med school, and therefore requires an enormous amount of preparation. I won't sugar-coat this one: for Step 1, you will likely study longer, more intensely, and more diligently than you ever have before. Years one and two of med school are challenging and rigorous, but Step 1 studying takes it to a whole new level due to the sheer volume of information and the relatively high pressure on this exam.

During my era of training, Step 1 was a scored exam. As previously mentioned, it was the single most important factor determining the strength of your residency application. It was often a very stressful experience because the Step 1 score was such a large determinant of a student's ability to match into their chosen specialty. Without an adequate score, students would potentially be unable to match into competitive specialties, which could limit their career choices. Though not everyone strives for these competitive specialties (orthopedics, neurosurgery, plastic surgery, dermatology to name a few), this did not diminish the importance and emotional magnitude of Step 1 for all of us. For every student this exam carried considerable weight and implications for the future, and therefore the pressure was high. But as mentioned prior, things have changed in terms of USMLE exam scoring. Step 1 became a pass/fail exam as of 2022. This change was made in an effort to reduce the stress on medical students preparing for Step 1 and to encourage a more holistic approach to residency applications. While it has likely reduced stress levels to some degree, this change has also shifted more focus onto the USMLE Step 2 exam. We will discuss the details of this exam in the next section; but bear in mind now that the high stakes situation, with a large amount of weight placed on the Step 1 exam in my era, is now more the reality for Step 2 in the present day. Both these exams are undoubtedly challenging and crucial (they cover a huge amount of material and must be passed to practice as a physician), but Step 2 now carries the most weight.

For me, Step 1 was an unprecedented time of intensity and stress which I do not look back upon fondly, if I am being honest. At UCSD, where I attended med school, we were given a six-week dedicated period just to study for this exam, free of any scheduled coursework. I (along with most of my peers) spent the majority of each day studying mountains of material, essentially reviewing everything we had learned in years one and two of med school. I had one study partner who I worked with closely, my good friend whom I thank to this day for being by my side throughout that grueling process. We both studied about ten to twelve hours per day, six to seven days per week during our dedicated study period. We scheduled each day of the six-week period far in advance, outlining which topics and lectures we would cover, basically down to the hour. We even scheduled time to eat, exercise, and a bit of time to relax. It may sound a bit excessive, but for most of us this level of detailed preparation was necessary to cover the tremendous amount of material we had to master for the exam. In addition to relearning countless concepts such as endocrine or neurologic physiology and memorizing innumerable facts like bacterial causes of infection and the antibiotics to treat them, we also spent hours working through hundreds of sample test questions. Much like the SAT and MCAT, the USMLE exams have a particular question style and there is considerable strategy that can be employed to effectively handle them. We needed to master a huge amount of material while developing the test-taking speed and skills required to succeed on this behemoth of a test. I have never studied harder and more consistently in my life than I did during my dedicated Step 1 study period. It ultimately paid off, as I learned a huge amount and succeeded on the exam; but it was a mental and physical grind which I certainly would not care to repeat.

I divulge these tough details not to discourage or strike fear in future medical students, but to be honest and avoid misleading readers. Step 1 and 2 will be times of significant learning but also stress. Studying for these exams will require serious perseverance and fortitude. I think I speak for many, if not all, of my colleagues when I say that we were very happy to put the USMLE exams in our rearview mirror. But with diligence and the same work ethic that got you this far, you will make it through and the feeling of accomplishment will be huge. Year two of medical school will culminate with the completion of Step 1, leading into the next stage of medical training: clinical rotations!

Medical School Year Three

Over the course of years three and four of medical school, students will complete rotations in the key clinical specialties: internal medicine, pediatrics, psychiatry, surgery, obstetrics/gynecology (OB/GYN), family medicine, and neurology. Each rotation typically lasts between one and three months (depending on the school and specialty) and is followed by a "shelf exam," which is essentially a final exam for that rotation. Shelf exams consist of 110 multiple choice questions to be completed in 165 minutes[3]. Grades in medical school clinical rotations are based on performance evaluations by supervising physicians as well as shelf exam scores, and typically fall into the following categories: honors, near honors, pass, and fail. In addition to daily clinical shifts, students will study for these exams throughout the rotation, which makes for a challenging schedule for third- and fourth-year med students.

Rotations themselves will occur at various hospitals or clinics, usually those affiliated with the medical school. Each rotation will have some inpatient time spent working on the hospital wards and some outpatient time spent working in clinics. Medical students will be part of a team, working alongside residents and attending physicians. Students will see patients mostly independently (sometimes with direct supervision though), and subsequently discuss the cases and formulate their treatment plans with the supervising resident/attending. During procedural rotations, students will often assist with procedures and surgeries. On surgical rotations specifically, students will spend hours in the operating room each day assisting with surgeries, being quizzed on topics such as anatomy or different surgical approaches and learning how to suture and perform other basic surgical techniques.

As you might guess, third year of med school can be exhilarating. It is the first opportunity a med student has to truly perform what they set out to do: provide meaningful care to real, live patients. The exposure to new situations and learning opportunities is unprecedented, making this an undoubtedly exciting time. On the flip side, this novel experience comes with its fair share of stress and challenges. I have always said that being a third-year medical student is akin to having a new job every four to six weeks (the interval at which students rotate to a new hospital or clinic setting). Each time a med student starts to gain some comfort and perhaps even proficiency, they are whisked off to the next rotation, often in a different hospital or medical specialty. They must start from square one again, learning the ins and outs of a brand new field of medicine. It is therefore difficult to get a real footing, and the med student is often left feeling like a perpetual novice. This is an unfortunate yet unavoidable aspect of being a medical student. Part of our growth in this role is seeing and experiencing each medical specialty first-hand; this requires working several different jobs from the ground up, starting anew each time. Dealing with this vast exposure is challenging, but it is what creates the broad foundation of medical knowledge that later leads to expertise. Furthermore, it is what allows students to choose their specialty; without exposure to each field of medicine, one could never truly decide on their path within this complex career. The experience of a third-year med student is equal parts stress and excitement, but one thing is for sure: it will be unforgettable.

I recall two very different third-year rotations vividly, the disparate experiences again representing the duality of life in the medical field. First was a rotation which I expected I would enjoy but did not end up taking a liking to: orthopedic surgery. On my three-month surgery rotation, I spent one month working in orthopedics at the hospital, assisting with an array of cases and surgeries, many of which dealt with trauma and significant injuries to bones and joints. I had pursued the field medicine years back with the notion that orthopedics would be a great fit for me. This is because my own first experience with the medical system occurred when I tore a ligament in my knee and needed orthopedic surgery to fix it, as mentioned earlier in Chapter 4. The impact my surgeon and therapists had on me can't fully be put into words. They helped me get back to basketball again. In a sense, they gave me my life back.

I was a huge sports fan (as I am to this day), and thus I expected my own experience with surgery and my passion for sports to translate into an interest in orthopedics. But interestingly, I was completely mistaken. Relatively early on in med school, I started to notice that I enjoyed medical specialties more than surgical ones. Although I did enjoy doing procedures, I did not love them. I preferred learning about physiology, thinking about complex medical problems, diagnosing patients with mysterious presentations, and creating treatment plans for those challenging cases. In other words, I enjoyed the cerebral aspect of internal medicine and did not fall in love with the physical skills needed to be an expert surgeon.

Now I must say, I have tremendous respect for surgeons and what they do. The precision with which they practice, the almost nonexistent room for error when performing intricate procedures, the physical fortitude it takes to execute long and complex surgeries—these are all extremely challenging skills which surgeons must perfect. They are also very intelligent (of course) and apply their cerebral approach to clinical care in a different manner. What I learned over the years, though, was that I enjoyed the mental approach of internal medicine, and the interpersonal aspect that goes with diagnosing and treating patients at the bedside, more than I enjoyed performing surgeries.

So back to my month as a third-year medical student on orthopedic surgery. Though I was discovering that my initial expectation to love "ortho" (as we call it) was perhaps misguided, I still did my very best to excel on this rotation. It is our responsibility as med students and future stewards of medical care to learn as much as we can at each opportunity. I was paired with one other medical student for this month. As the lowest on the totem pole in terms of skill and experience, it was our job to arrive first every morning and perform a relatively straightforward task: preparing a list of all patients admitted on the orthopedics service. Simple enough. Each morning, we would curate the patients' vital signs, labs, imaging studies, and other results into a centralized list. This list would then be used by the team of residents (led by the chief resident) to do rapid-fire "rounds," which is when the team would examine the patients and formulate a plan for the day.

The most joyous part of the experience was that rounds began at the (completely normal) hour of 5:30 AM. This meant that my compadre and I needed to have the list prepared and the patient information ready by that time. We quickly realized that we had to reach the hospital no later than 4:30 AM to make this happen. We served a simple albeit important function to the team and we did it to the best of our ability, trying to learn as much as possible and of course impress our supervisors along the way. But the pain of those morning is something I still remember to this day: waking up at 3:30 AM six days a week, quickly getting ready and leaving my house by 4:00 AM in pitch-black darkness, driving to the hospital in essentially the dead of night to begin a long day of work. It was a physical grind. After rounds, we spent long hours in the hospital, assisting with surgeries and seeing new patients on the floors throughout the day.

The funny thing is, it was only such a grind for me and my med student companion because neither of us loved surgery. It was still very important that we be there, that we learn the broad skills of suturing, surgical techniques, and how to manage orthopedic injuries and traumas. But we knew that ultimately, orthopedics (and surgery in general) was not for us. Each day we learned as much as we could, as was our duty. There were certainly fun moments, but it was not at all an easy experience. The sheer physical toll of the hours, not to mention studying for the surgery shelf exam and the stress of impressing a demanding set of supervising surgeons, made the experience a challenge.

Ironically, some of my best friends in medical school absolutely loved orthopedics, doing the same rotation and finding it fascinating. They ultimately ended up pursuing ortho as a career, and practice as orthopedic surgeons today. This is one of the interesting things about medicine that represents its broad and diverse nature, which we have discussed before: we all start in the same place in medical school, but based on our personal preferences and interests, we end up in vastly different specialties with completely unique skillsets.

It is important to keep this in mind when thinking about your intended specialty within the world of medicine. We all learn so much along that way that is more likely than not that our preferences will change. That is completely okay. Keeping an open mind and being generous with yourself as you explore your passions is important when selecting both a specialty and a career. Now that brings me back to my original statement about two disparate rotations which I clearly recall from third year of medical school. Once I realized that surgery was not quite right for me, I gravitated more and more to internal medicine, and particularly inpatient hospital medicine, which is what I do today. I rotated for two months on inpatient medicine services in the major hospitals affiliated with my medical school. In the internal medicine world, I felt much more at home. I truly enjoyed seeing patients with all kinds of medical maladies as mentioned earlier, from heart failure to liver failure, cancers to blood clots, kidney disorders to mysteries of infectious disease. The pace—medically managing lots of patients while doing shorter procedures, allowing a bit more time to sit and speak with patients and think critically about their cases—this appealed to my personal preferences much more closely.

There was certainly still plenty of stress, as I was learning on the job and so many skills were brand new and therefore uncomfortable. One particularly memorable way that the stress in medical school manifests is when students are asked questions and expected to answer in a public format, in front of their peers and other medical providers. This practice has historically been called "pimping," although this term and its negative connotations have fallen out of favor for obvious reasons. In essence, this practice employs the Socratic method of teaching, which is used in much of the clinical education in medical school and residency. Named for the Greek philosopher Socrates who developed it, the Socratic method is an approach by which the teacher asks questions of the students in order to probe their understanding of a topic and find potential gaps in their knowledge, which can be improved with additional teaching[4]. This approach in and of itself is not a bad one; it makes sense for practical education in the hospital or clinics when seeing patients in real clinical scenarios. But it can take on a more malignant form, when students are put on the spot and embarrassed in front of their colleagues, perhaps as a method of teaching a memorable lesson they will not forget. This more aggressive form of the Socratic method should be avoided, as it can engender a culture of fear. If medical students are not comfortable speaking up and asking questions, they may not ask for help when they truly need it. I am a firm believer that a truly safe teaching environment, one in which students feel comfortable seeking support and advice from their supervisors, is essential when learning to care for human lives. But it is important to know that, although imperfect, some degree of the Socratic teaching method does exist in the medical education system. You will certainly encounter it during your time as a medical student and resident. The best approach is to use these instances as learning opportunities rather than intimidating moments—to maintain humility but also not be afraid to speak up, answer to the best of your ability, and (most importantly) ask questions.

I remember several instances when I was subject to this mode of questioning as a medical student on my third- and fourth-year rotations. I often learned something valuable, but admit that sometimes this process created additional stress which was probably unnecessary. Despite these moments, I did very much enjoy my third-year rotation on the internal medicine wards. Amidst the challenging moments, I had many great experiences and memorable patient encounters. My clinical skills and medical knowledge grew quickly. I met mentors in the form of residents and attending physicians, role models who I could see myself emulating one day. Ultimately, I felt at home and knew that if I pursued internal medicine, something within that field would be a good fit for me. I was right—today I happily practice as an internal medicine hospitalist. I trace the early moments of finding my place as a physician back to my third year of med school. This year will be an unprecedented time of learning and growth and will set you on the path to your future career.

Medical School Year Four

Early in year four of medical school, students will take Step 2 of the USMLE. This test is a bit different from its predecessor Step 1. Prior to 2020, it consisted of two separate testing days: Step 2 Clinical Knowledge (CK) and Step 2 Clinical Skills (CS). The second component, Step 2 CS, was a clinical skills exam consisting of several observed/graded clinical encounters with standardized patients played by actors. In May 2020, with the arrival of the COVID-19 pandemic, Step 2 CS was put on hold. In early 2021, Step 2 CS was discontinued altogether, with plans to revamp the exam and launch a new version in the future.

As of now, medical students only need to complete one portion of this exam in fourth year of medical school: Step 2

CK. It consists of a maximum of 318 questions in a multiple-choice format very similar to Step 1. The exam focuses more heavily on clinical scenarios rather than basic science/theory which comprise a considerable portion of Step 1. It is a nine-hour exam divided into eight blocks with a maximum of forty questions each[5]. As mentioned prior, Step 2 scores are a crucial component of the residency application process. This exam has a numerical score and is not pass/fail as Step 1 is now; therefore, Step 2 carries much more weight than it used to. Although the transition was very recent (Step 1 became pass/fail in 2022) and objective data is lacking, many say Step 2 is becoming the most important exam in medical school with the strongest influence on residency application strength and the student's ability to match. Personally, my experience preparing for Step 2 was challenging, but considerably less stressful than Step 1. For the current generation of medical students, this experience may be flipped (or the two exams may be equally challenging) due to the change in scoring and relative weight of each exam.

Year four will then continue very similarly to year three with students completing the remaining clinical rotations in the core clinical specialties mentioned prior. Students will then complete key rotations in the field(s) that they are considering applying to for residency. These rotations function as a kind of "test-run," or a sample of what the life of a resident in that specialty will be like. The fourth-year students will be given more responsibility but also closely evaluated, with performance reviews from supervisors playing an important role in their eventual residency application.

Med students will apply for residency in their chosen specialty during the first half of fourth year. Just like undergrad transitioning into med school, this time will be the culmination of four years of hard work but will require some work itself. The residency application consists primarily of the following, in a rough descending order of importance[6]:

1. USMLE Scores (Step 1 and Step 2)
2. Letters of recommendation
3. Medical Student Performance Evaluation (MSPE) – also known as the Dean's letter, this is a written summary of the student's performance in the core clinical rotations during med school. Although not a "report card" per se, this is influenced by clerkship grades and also contains quotes from performance reviews during rotations.
4. Personal statement
5. Grades in Medical School Clerkships
6. Extracurricular activities

Luckily, only one application needs to be submitted to all programs and there is no secondary application for residency. Once the above materials have been submitted (typically by early fall), students will be invited for interviews with residency programs. Although residency interviews were traditionally completed in person so that candidates could experience the program first-hand, since the COVID-19 pandemic, the vast majority of residency interviews are now completed virtually[7]. Regardless, the interview process is a chance for programs to make their final decisions on applicants and for applicants to learn about and closely evaluate their selected residency program. Applicants typically complete around ten interviews per specialty (sometimes more and occasionally students apply to multiple specialties, increasing their number of applications/interviews). Again, the cost of interviews and travel is covered by the applicant and not the program, but this burden is considerably lower currently based on the prevalence of virtual interviews. Nonetheless, interviews are a great opportunity to increase exposure to training/practice differences at institutions across the country.

A unique component of the residency application process, one which you may have heard of but perhaps may not completely understand, is The Match. The Match refers to a system by which medical students applying to residency are matched to only one program in the specialty of their choosing, rather than receiving multiple acceptances from which they can select one program to attend (as occurs in most traditional application processes). How does The Match work? It is based on a complex computer algorithm. I would be unable to explain its intricacies, but the take-home points are as follows:

Students apply to a number of residency programs and receive interview invitations to some of those programs. After completing interviews, applicants rank as many programs as they would like in order of their personal preference. They then submit this "rank list" from which they will be matched to only one program (or occasionally and unfortunately, none at all). Meanwhile, residency programs will interview dozens to hundreds of applicants (depending on the size of the program) for a designated number of residency spots. Programs will then rank each of the applicants in order of the program's preference, also submitting a rank list when this is complete. The algorithm will then take both applicant and program preferences into account and match each student to just one program, as high as possible on the students rank list.

The Match system is designed to match as many students as possible to as high a choice as possible and leave the fewest number of residency spots open/unmatched. Unfortunately, a small minority of students do not match to any program. In 2022, 92.9% of US fourth-year MD students matched into residency positions, while 91.3% of US DO students matched[8]. Those who do not match have three options: 1) utilize a system called SOAP (Supplemental Offer and Acceptance Program) which opens unmatched positions for which applicants can publicly apply, and in effect "scramble" into an unfilled residency slot[9]; 2) apply again through the Match for their preferred residency position the following year; or 3) pivot to an alternative, non-clinical career which does not require residency training. As the numbers show, not matching into a residency position is relatively uncommon. It is more of a risk in the most competitive specialties such as orthopedic surgery, neurosurgery, and plastic surgery for example. Do not fear this outcome though. Stay positive, as with hard work and preparation throughout medical school, you are very likely to succeed in The Match process.

The Match does come with the unique stress of not knowing which program you will attend until a specific day, called Match Day. This occurs in March of fourth year of medical school and is the day on which all students find out their "Match", or the result of their application. Once a student matches into a program, he or she is essentially bound to that program and typically does not have the flexibility to go elsewhere. There is some beauty in the simplicity of matching to just one program, but also some inherent stress that comes with the applicant's lack of autonomy and flexibility in choosing their final destination. For most, Match Day is an exciting moment, a positive culmination and celebration of all the hard work required to reach residency.

Once Match Day is complete, you are essentially on the last couple holes of the back nine of medical school. Most students finish up a last rotation or two in the spring prior to graduation in June. Residency training then starts in late June or early July, depending on the program. Many medical students have the opportunity to take some vacation time in May and/or June of their fourth year of medical school in order to recharge prior to beginning residency. I personally was able to travel internationally at the end of my fourth year, as did many of my peers. I always look back on this time very fondly; it was a much-needed break prior to starting residency, one which really rejuvenated my spirit. Put simply, it was one of the best times of my life. The beat goes on in terms of medical training and clinical practice, so it is important to take these opportunities to rest, replenish, and recharge before moving on to the next step of the journey: residency!

Chapter 10: What is Residency Really Like?

And just like that, the marathon that is medical education and training continues on. It really is a long-distance race, won on stamina and grit much more than speed or show. At this point in the twenty-six-mile race, you are somewhere around the midway point or slightly beyond, depending on the length of your residency. If completing a three-year residency, you are certainly past mile thirteen, having achieved eight years of academic success preceding this moment. If you are pursuing something like neurosurgery or interventional cardiology, which can require eight years of combined residency/fellowship training, you are approaching the midway point of your journey.

Regardless, you have achieved a whole lot thus far, and that is to be commended. With that said, you have plenty left to go! As mentioned in Chapter 9, there is not much truth to the statement that getting into medical school "is the hard part." Each step poses unique challenges and incites unique growth. Residency (and fellowship if you choose to pursue it) will be perhaps the most challenging and rigorous; but I would contend that for this very reason, it is the time of greatest growth from a personal, educational, and professional standpoint. You will likely work harder than ever before and encounter numerous high-stress, high-intensity situations. But you will also experience great triumphs and emerge a well-trained, battle-tested physician. Residency is when you truly gain the expertise of medical practice which only experience can produce. Like coal turning to diamond, through immense pressure you will emerge as what you always imagined becoming: a full-fledged, independently practicing physician.

The Lingo: Types of Medical Trainees and Professionals

Before discussing the training that occurs after med school, which in the medical world is referred to as "postgraduate training," it is prudent to discuss the lingo associated with residency (and fellowship). Medicine has a confusing nomenclature because the terms do not necessarily mean what they do in other spheres of life. Let's discuss these terms now to establish a clear understanding of the different roles played in medical training and practice.

Intern

First, the most confusing title of all medical professionals: *intern*. What is an intern? Set aside all the associations you normally ascribe to this word in the business world or elsewhere. In medicine, an intern means a first-year resident physician, plain and simple. That means that every single resident and attending physician was once an intern; we all had to go through first year of residency and thus we all held this title at some point. This title has nothing to do with the commonly held definitions of an intern (like someone working a summer job to buff up their resume or an unpaid position at a company—though ironically, medical interns/residents also do not make much money). Rather, *intern* in the medical world is simply the designation held during the first year of residency training. During this time, the trainee develops the bread-and-butter skills needed for the practice of medicine, primarily under the tutelage of their more seasoned peers (residents).

It is important to note that an intern (and every subsequent designation that follows) is already a physician. Anyone who has graduated from medical school and obtained the MD or DO degree is in fact a full-fledged physician, and they have earned that title. The difference is that until completing internship, residency, and the steps that may follow, physicians typically cannot practice medicine independently. Therefore interns, residents, and fellows are physicians who care for patients on a daily basis with considerable skill and knowledge—they simply have not completed full training in their chosen specialty, and thus are not yet independent practitioners of medicine.

Resident

Next comes what is likely a more familiar term to most: *resident*. Though this is the overarching term for all medical trainees who enter residency after medical school, the specific job title of *resident* is actually assumed after the first year of residency (a.k.a. internship) is complete. Thus, residents are those who are in residency training from year two and onwards, sometimes continuing for up to six or even eight years in certain surgical specialties. Residents function as team leaders supervising interns and less experienced residents, while working in close conjunction with the attending physician (more on this designation in a moment). The resident is the physician you have observed closely in pop-culture shows such as *Grey's Anatomy* or *Scrubs* (though the experience is obviously quite different from what is portrayed on TV). Residents are the backbone workforce of academic training hospitals, such as your local university hospital, performing much of the day-to-day patient care.

Fellow

The next designation in the hierarchy of medical training is the *fellow*. They may or may not be jolly-good, as the *fellow* is again a term with a unique medical definition that most are not familiar with. A fellow is a physician completing further training beyond residency in a chosen area of specialization. Fellowships can be completed in subspecialties after any kind of residency, including internal medicine, surgery, pediatrics, and so on. A fellow has already completed residency in one of these fields. Instead of choosing to start career practice, a fellow has elected to pursue more subspecialty training. For example, a resident who has completed three years of internal medicine residency can pursue a fellowship in cardiology, which will be three additional years of training. They will again work in hospitals and clinics year-round learning the broad array of skills necessary to practice as a cardiologist. Often, they will also conduct research in their chosen field, cultivating this skill and contributing to their specialty's body of knowledge. Once the fellow completes cardiology training, they can start their independent career practice or choose to pursue yet another sub-fellowship in something like interventional cardiology or electrophysiology. Ultimately, in each field there comes a point when no further fellowship training is available, but you get the idea. Fellows are those who have completed residency but have chosen to train further in order to gain more specialized expertise before officially starting their independent career as an attending.

Attending

Finally, there is the ultimate step and clinical designation in the career of a physician: *attending*. Again, this is a term which is specific to medicine. The attending is the physician who has completed all their medical training (meaning at least residency and possibly fellowship as well) and has begun their independent medical practice. Attendings are fully trained physicians who have reached the end of the long road that is medical education. They can work in a number of different practice settings, including academic institutions overseeing a team of medical students, interns, residents, and/or fellows or non-teaching institutions treating their own patients rather than supervising trainees. Many options exist within the world of independent medical practice, but one thing is for sure: once you are an attending physician, you've made it. You have reached the peak of the mountain of medical education and training. One day many of the readers of this book will reach this coveted position. I hope the knowledge you gain from these pages will help you along the way!

Now that we have established the medical lingo necessary to understand the stages of medical training, let's delve into what the experience is actually like. Let me start by saying that the nuanced experiences of various residencies may differ considerably based upon specialty; for example, pediatrics versus general surgery will offer very different experiences, each with their own benefits and challenges. Therefore, in reading this chapter, it is important to understand that what is stated here certainly does not capture all the broad experiences of residency training. Despite my effort to depict a comprehensive experience, my accounts will inevitably be somewhat biased toward my own personal path. But across specialties there are some common strokes—shared themes, experiences, and emotions which we all encounter. I have synthesized these patterns based on my experiences and the many conversations I have had with countless friends in other medical and surgical specialties, creating as cohesive a picture as possible.

Most students starting medical school do not truly understand what life as a resident entails. And yet residency makes up a huge portion of the journey. It is the crux of the experience which molds a student into a physician, healer, and practitioner of medicine. The insight that follows will make you much more equipped to decide if medicine is right for you, and much more prepared to succeed when you do make that decision.

Residency Year One: Internship

As discussed, intern year is the start of residency training and the true beginning of a physician's clinical practice. There are technically two different buckets into which intern years are categorized: the "categorical" year, when the intern year and residency years are completed in the same specialty (such as internal medicine, pediatrics, or general surgery); and the "preliminary" or "transitional" year, when the initial internship year is completed before moving on to a residency in a different specialty. A preliminary year or transitional year is required for certain residencies such as anesthesiology, dermatology, neurology, and radiology, to name a few[1]. The preliminary year and transitional years differ slightly. A preliminary intern year is either completed in internal medicine or surgery, before moving onto a field with overlapping skills/knowledge with either of those specialties. The transitional intern year, on the other hand, is a broad overview during which the intern rotates through many different specialties of medicine, and then moves on to another residency field. There are nuances to each of these options, but the majority of graduating medical students pursue categorical internships/residencies, unless they choose one of the aforementioned specialties which require either a preliminary or transitional year. The final detail to note is that an intern pursuing a preliminary or transitional year will need to apply separately to secure this spot during The Match. They may actually complete this year at a different institution than their eventual residency program.

Now that we have established the different types of intern years, what does the experience actually look and feel like? Intern year is simultaneously one of the most daunting *and* exciting steps on the road to becoming a physician. It is a whirlwind year, an absolute blur of learning and skillset expansion unlike any other. Interns begin their year working under the supervision of residents, who have already completed anywhere from one to seven years of residency training. Interns are the first line of medical care for patients in both the hospital and clinic. They evaluate and examine patients directly, creating treatment plans which they then discuss and alter as needed with the help of the supervising resident or attending. They then deliver medical care in the form of medications and procedures, and perform documentation of what they have done (in other words, they treat patients and write notes!). This care occurs in both inpatient (in the hospital) and outpatient (in the clinic) settings; but for many specialties, the majority of intern year and residency itself are spent working within the hospital. For example, internal medicine and surgical residencies tend to have an inpatient focus, and thus the majority of the time is spent in the emergency room, medical wards, and operating rooms of the hospital. Incidentally, interns and residents used to spend so much time working in the hospital (and often still do) that they were referred to as "housestaff." This name and the term "resident" literally stem from the fact that these trainees spent the majority of their time working and even residing within the hospital (the house). We often refer to patients admitted to the hospital as "in house." In many ways, during residency and even beyond, the hospital becomes a home away from home for medical trainees. Times have changed somewhat, and residents do have slightly better hours and more time outside the hospital than they did many years ago. But the general theme has not deviated too far from its origin: interns and residents work long hours, spending the majority of their lives in their new home (the hospital) with their new family (their co-interns and residents).

Inpatient Life

Let's first focus on the intern's inpatient experience as this typically comprises the lion's share of the first year of residency, with the exception of some outpatient-focused residencies (such as family medicine). Recall that it is difficult to generalize as there are differences across specialties, in particular between surgical and medical fields. Typically, though, an intern's life looks something like this.

Interns work as part of a team under direct supervision of residents and more peripheral supervision of attendings. Interns themselves supervise and teach third- and fourth-year medical students who are also part of the team, though more of that educational responsibility lies with the resident. The intern is responsible for a certain number of the hospitalized patients on the team's inpatient service. For example, interns in internal medicine residency typically are responsible for caring for and "rounding on" eight to ten patients per day. These patients are the direct responsibility of the intern, who examines them, writes orders, performs procedures, and finally writes notes. Though the resident assists the intern with these tasks and teaches throughout, the intern is the first line of medical treatment and primarily responsible for these patients most of the time.

Interns typically arrive quite early, between 5:00 AM and 7:00 AM in most cases, and "pre-round" on their patients. This means that they look up all necessary data (overnight hospital events, vital signs, morning lab values, imaging, etc.) and subsequently examine the patient. Throughout this process, the intern synthesizes the new data to formulate a plan of care for each patient that day, which they will present to the team on "rounds." Rounds are the formal process during which the whole team sees each patient to discuss the plan and provide education to junior members of the team. This process is quite variable in different specialties; for example, rounds are typically much faster on a surgical service to allow more time for the operating room. During parts of the day, the team will be responsible for new admissions entering the hospital from the emergency room, and the interns will admit new patients during those hours. Procedures that need to be performed will typically be done later in the day if non-urgent, or immediately if emergent.

Time spent doing procedures versus time spent medically managing patients on the hospital floors is where the experience of the surgical intern will differ from that of the medical intern. Though most of the operating room experience in surgery residency occurs in years two and onward, surgical interns will spend some time in the operating room in addition to learning how to care for the pre- and post-operative patients on the hospital floors. Meanwhile medical interns (and residents) will do some procedures at the bedside, but the majority of their work will be management of patients throughout the hospital with medications and non-surgical treatments. It is important to note that all the while, interns, residents, and attendings across specialties work collaboratively. It is relatively uncommon these days that any hospitalized patient has one single issue requiring only one treatment team. Internal medicine or pediatric physicians, surgeons, and specialists all collaborate to provide patients whatever specialty care they need. There is plenty of crosstalk between specialties, again representing how medicine truly is a team sport.

Another specialty which has a unique experience based on the nature of its work is emergency medicine. Emergency interns will see patients on shifts mostly in the emergency room; some patients will be treated and sent home from the ER and some will be admitted to the hospital with the help of the inpatient teams. Emergency medicine interns and residents will perform various procedures throughout the day according to each patient's needs. They will develop the broad skillset needed to stabilize and preliminarily treat most medical issues which walk through the door, subsequently moving patients on to the right specialty service when they need further care.

Interns work shifts like these on average six days per week, generally ten to twelve (or more) hours per day. This often amounts to eighty-hour work weeks (or more, once again). It is no secret that interns work hard in the pursuit of medical skills and knowledge. Interns and residents alike must be ready to commit themselves fully to their work, as the hours and effort required are certainly demanding. It can be difficult to handle such an intense workload and maintain balance in life. I find that most trainees discover what non-medical outlets are best for them during medical school—whether it be exercising, reading, or spending time with family and friends—and continue to employ those strategies during residency. But the time pressure and demands are certainly higher during intern year and residency than ever before. I will be honest that during my internship/residency, I certainly sacrificed plenty of the personal time that I longed to spend exercising, playing basketball, or relaxing with friends and family. This is inevitably part of the process. But each individual must strive for professional growth, while striking enough balance to maintain happiness outside of the hospital. It is no easy task, and it will be something each intern must navigate in their own way.

Outpatient Life

The day-to-day outpatient experience of the intern is quite different from the inpatient world. The model of work/education does not change, though: interns continue to evaluate patients, summarizing and presenting a treatment plan to a supervising doctor (typically an attending), and delivering medical care to the patient. But the schedule, experience, and demands of the job are quite different in the outpatient setting. On clinic weeks/months, which are less frequent than inpatient time for most internships/residencies, interns work five days per week and have weekends off. This provides a nice respite from the sometimes brutal grind that can be inpatient training. In clinic, interns are responsible for a subset of patients who arrive for scheduled appointments. They evaluate the patients and present a plan to the attending prior to enacting the plan and writing their notes. Writing notes is a crucial skill that all physicians must develop. The practice starts in medical school and continues in residency, such that the graduating resident knows how to efficiently document all necessary medical information. Notes vary in style and format between providers and across specialties, but typically cover three basic areas: "subjective," a recounting of the patients reported symptoms; "objective," a summary of objective data including vital signs, exam findings, lab results, and imaging; and "assessment/plan," the physician's synthesis of the raw data into a diagnosis and treatment plan.

In specialties such as internal or family medicine, interns and residents also treat their own panel of primary care patients on a continuous basis. Throughout their entire training, these interns and residents act as the true primary care physician for these patients. This is a great experience and an opportunity for trainees to take ownership of their patients' health, establishing continuity and longevity in these relationships. Some residencies, such as family medicine and psychiatry, are primarily based in the outpatient setting, as this is the predominant location of practice for attendings in those fields. Each residency will have a different composition of inpatient and outpatient time based on the educational demands and skills needed to practice effectively in that field.

With the great variety of physician specialties, there are nuances to each intern role. But the patterns and descriptions we covered will provide a general framework to understand what an intern's life in the hospital is typically like. As you move forward in your career and gain more exposure, you will also gain more perspective on the life of an intern in your specific field of interest. Reflecting on my experience, my most memorable month of intern year was my first inpatient internal medicine rotation. It was at the local county hospital, which served many of San Diego's uninsured patients in need, those who didn't have the means to afford their own medical care. The hospital was and still is an amazing place to practice and learn, with remarkable disease pathology and tons of opportunity to truly help patients. But it was not necessarily the most glamorous place to work, as few county hospitals are. We worked out of somewhat rudimentary rooms with limited space, teeming with medical students, interns, and residents alike. We all scrounged for time and space as we were busy learning to manage several complex patients, many of which had new and exciting diseases we had never treated before. We would arrive early and examine our patients, reading up on the diseases that were less familiar and formulating our plans before rounds with our supervising attending. Later in the day we would dash to the ER to treat patients with alcohol withdrawal, methamphetamine intoxication, or bloodstream infections in the setting of HIV/AIDS. The amount of learning was immense. These were difficult but exciting times which I will never forget. This was also the hospital in which I so memorably severed my finger while performing my first procedure on a patient (remember Chapter 1?). I did this all alongside an awesome group of co-interns. We bonded quickly, much as sports teams do when experiencing both adversity and excitement together. Some of those interns are still among my closest friends today. We grew up together. We became physicians together. No matter how challenging it may have been, it was an awesome time of personal growth and interpersonal connection. These are memories I will always cherish.

Residency Year Two and Beyond

After moving on from intern year, the trainee gains the next title on the road of physician life: *resident*. Resident life structurally bears many similarities to intern life. It follows a similar daily schedule and inpatient bias (for most fields), with perhaps a slight increase in outpatient rotations compared to intern year. For those specialties which are more outpatient focused, there may be a large amount of outpatient rotations with each subsequent year of residency. For many specialties though, the focus remains on work within the hospital. In surgical residencies, each year typically offers more time in the operating room, as thousands of hours are needed to master the skills necessary to be a safe and effective surgeon. In specialties which provide some procedural care, such as internal medicine or emergency medicine, resident years are also spent performing and perfecting procedures and then educating interns/junior residents on how to perform them as well ("do one" and "teach one").

Aside from these differences among specialties, many of the components of resident life mirror that of the intern but from a step above, with greater responsibility and less oversight. On inpatient teams, residents typically become the team leader, responsible for each patient and the supervision/education of the med students and interns. For example, on an inpatient internal medicine service, the resident will usually oversee two interns and two to three medical students. The team will typically care for somewhere between fifteen and twenty patients per day. While the interns handle only their own eight to ten patients, the resident is responsible for intimately understanding all twenty. The resident will do less of the day-to-day examination and patient care at the bedside but will need to review all the data and know the patients and treatment plans in even more depth/detail than the interns. The resident is responsible for reviewing the interns' and med students' work, ensuring that patients are being cared for appropriately and making sure that important components of care are not missed. For example, before or after rounds, the resident might identify a nuance of disease management that was overlooked and provide education to the interns and med students on how to implement this care. As we will discuss in the following chapter, the academic attending does much the same job as the resident with yet another level of review, using their greater experience and expertise to ensure that patients are being cared for skillfully and safely.

The resident will typically lead rounds each day in conjunction with the attending. New patient admissions will be completed by the interns with the help of the resident. Thus, the resident is the core of the team, making sure the interns are supported and the attending gets the necessary information. Another key component of a resident's job is medical student/intern education. Residents provide on-the-go teaching throughout the day as needed, as well as small formal lectures on key educational topics. Learning to be an effective educator is a large portion of the resident role, and this is reflected in their daily life. Residents are required to conduct educational lectures for larger groups within the residency program to educate their peers and develop their own teaching skills. Many residents also complete research projects in an area of interest, some of which they will present at research conferences and ultimately publish in journals. Education, public speaking, and team leadership are a large component of resident life, in conjunction with the continued mastery of medical knowledge and surgical skill.

Both interns and residents will typically rotate through multiple inpatient units, all of which have a different function and thus require unique education. Residents of most specialties typically spend time rotating in the emergency room, medical/surgical wards, and the intensive care unit (ICU). Depending on the type of residency, the amount of time spent in each of these settings will vary based on the level of skill and proficiency required for practice in that field.

Let's take my experience as an internal medicine resident for example, to help illustrate how residency can actually play out. My training was three years long, which is the normal length for specialties such as internal medicine, pediatrics, and family medicine. During my intern year, I spent about five months rotating on the general internal medicine wards, three months in the ICU, one month in the ER, and two months in subspecialty or primary care clinics, with a few weeks left for vacation. During my time as a resident (years two and three), I had a similar split with slightly more outpatient months (three to four per year) and slightly fewer inpatient months (seven to eight per year). In years two and three though, I still spent a few months on the wards, two to three months in the ICU, and a few weeks in the ER. The remaining time was spent getting deeper exposure to subspecialties like cardiology, pulmonology, oncology, endocrinology, nephrology, and dermatology, usually in clinic settings but also sometimes in the hospital. This broad exposure is key, as the resident must gain proficiency and eventually skill managing any kind of disease which falls under the umbrella of their specialty. Our internal medicine residents also had the opportunity for some elective rotations with other specialties such as surgery, neurology, or psychiatry, depending on their personal interests. The experience became more diverse with each passing year as we were allowed to expand upon the bread-and-butter skills we had gained as an intern and receive more specialized training/education.

A Word on Fellowship

In the final year of residency, residents elect to either finish their training and apply for jobs/start their career practice or pursue additional fellowship training. We will review more on fellowship options in Chapter 11; but the idea, as previously mentioned, is that the physician can gain more subspecialized education with one to three more years of training. For example, a pulmonary critical care fellow will complete an additional three years of education and training after residency (which was usually three years of internal medicine or pediatrics). They will learn the skills of a full-fledged pulmonologist: working in ICUs alongside an attending or overseeing a team of residents, interns, and med students (as you can see there is a lot of teamwork in medicine); performing consultations on patients with pulmonary issues who are on the hospital wards; learning and perfecting procedures such as intubation, thoracentesis, bronchoscopy, and even endobronchial ultrasound (the details of these procedures are not important, but I mention them to illustrate the example of specialized fellowship skills); and working in clinics with patients who require pulmonary disease management. This pattern of gaining more detailed expertise in the specialty will be the model for all fellowships. One of the biggest components of some fellowships is learning new procedural skills. For example, surgical specialties such as orthopedics have fellowships in hand surgery or foot/ankle surgery; cardiologists can perform additional fellowships with more training on how to place a stent for a patient with a heart attack (interventional cardiology) or a pacemaker for someone with an abnormal heart rhythm (electrophysiology); anesthesiologists can get specialized training in pain management procedures; and so on and so forth.

Different "Flavors" of Residency Training

Though the residency Match system cannot boast quite as many flavors as Baskin-Robbins, there are many specialty options that graduating medical students can choose from, each with its own unique flavor. It is important to know that each of these options differs (quite significantly in some cases) in length and type of training. Each specialty will offer a very different experience, from the skills learned to the patients encountered. Knowing these options early in the process of considering a career in medicine is important; it arms you with an understanding of what your training and career may look and feel like, which is more knowledge than the vast majority of premeds have.

As I have discussed earlier and will continue to reiterate, knowledge is power. This notion is especially true in this circumstance. The commitment to residency is a huge one—in years, in effort, and in the toll it takes on you emotionally and physically. Therefore, it is only logical that students committing to the path of medicine should understand *in advance* what the commitment can entail and what their options will be within the field. Without this information, many are flying blind toward turbulent winds which invariably lie ahead. Though residency is an amazing experience which is necessary for physicians to gain expertise, it is both quite lengthy and quite challenging; therefore, it should be understood before it is embarked upon. Here are the different subspecialties which can be chosen after medical school, the typical length of training, and the type of work each is primarily comprised of.

1. Anesthesiology – four years (one year of preliminary training[i] followed by three years of anesthesiology). Primarily operating room and inpatient.
2. Emergency Medicine – three to four years. Primarily ER and inpatient.
3. Ear, Nose and Throat Surgery (also known as Otolaryngology) – five years. Inpatient, outpatient, and operating room.
4. Family Medicine – three years. Primarily outpatient with some inpatient.
5. General surgery[ii] – five years (sometimes with a sixth year of research). Inpatient, outpatient, and operating room.
6. Internal Medicine[iii] – three years. Both inpatient and outpatient (though more heavily inpatient).
7. Interventional Radiology (IR) – six to seven years total (one year of preliminary training followed by five years of integrated IR residency; or one year of preliminary training followed by four years of diagnostic radiology followed by two years if IR training). Early years spent in

---

i Preliminary training refers to either preliminary or transitional intern year, as discussed earlier in this chapter.

ii General surgery residency can be completed alone, after which the graduate can be an attending general surgeon. It can also be followed by a fellowship in subspecialties such as cardiothoracic surgery, colorectal surgery, pediatric surgery, transplant surgery, and vascular surgery (among others). These fellowships last one to three years.

iii Internal medicine and pediatrics residencies can be completed alone, after which the graduate can be an attending internist or pediatrician, typically practicing as either a primary care doctor (all outpatient) or a hospitalist (all inpatient). These residencies can also be followed by a fellowship in subspecialties such as allergy/immunology, cardiology, endocrinology, gastroenterology, nephrology, oncology, pulmonary critical care, and rheumatology (among others). These fellowships last two to three years.

radiology reading room examining images, followed by heavy procedural years, both inpatient and outpatient.

8. Neurology – four years (one year of preliminary training followed by three years of neurology). Inpatient and outpatient.

9. Neurosurgery – seven to eight years. Inpatient, outpatient, and operating room.

10. Obstetrics/Gynecology – four years. Inpatient, outpatient, and operating room.

11. Ophthalmology – four years (one year of preliminary training followed by three years of ophthalmology). Primarily outpatient and operating room, with some inpatient.

12. Orthopedic Surgery – five years (sometimes with a sixth year of research). Inpatient, outpatient, and operating room.

13. Pathology – four years. Primarily in the pathology lab examining body tissues (limited direct patient care).

14. Pediatrics – three years. Inpatient and outpatient (slightly more outpatient).

15. Physical Medicine and Rehabilitation – three to four years. Inpatient and outpatient.

16. Psychiatry – four years. Inpatient and outpatient (though more heavily outpatient).

17. Radiation Oncology – five years (one year of preliminary training followed by four years of radiation oncology). Primarily outpatient.

18. Radiology (also known as diagnostic radiology) – four years (one year of preliminary training followed by three years of

diagnostic radiology). Primarily in radiology reading room examining images (limited direct patient care).
19. Urology – five years. Inpatient, outpatient, and operating room.

The list above is quite detailed, likely above the scope of knowledge needed by an aspiring premed. But it serves three purposes for you as the reader: first, to inform you of the several options available for specialty training after med school; second, to provide you with a mental roadmap of the years required to complete training and the types of work different physicians can perform in their careers; and third, to help you appreciate the complexity and plethora of possibilities for specialization on the road to becoming an attending physician. This list is also not completely exhaustive. There are many additional fellowship training options which physicians can choose to gain additional expertise after residency (more on this in Chapter 11). What is most important, though, is appreciating that when you embark on the path to getting into medical school, you have only started the first step of the process. There are many remaining years of training to be completed and many decisions to be made about what suits you best in your career as a doctor. I found through my own experience and that of my peers, it was easy to become nearsighted and only focus on getting accepted to medical school. This in and of itself was such a daunting task that I found myself losing sight of what I really wanted out of it, and what my career plans might be after I got in. Keeping this bigger picture in mind and understanding the next steps after med school and beyond will make you a much more mature and prepared applicant to join the medical profession.

Ultimately, do not let the length of the process deter you if you have chosen medicine for the right reasons. It will all be worth it if a life as a physician is the right choice for you (think back to Chapters 4 and 5). Think of these steps and career branch points as opportunities rather than burdens. Medicine truly is a fascinating field, and you will have countless ways to satisfy your interests and passions along the way. With the knowledge above and the roadmap of your potential future after med school, you are vastly more equipped to understand the career of a physician and whether it is the right path for you.

What is the Emotional Impact of (Medical School and) Residency?

The emotional impact of medical education and training is a complex question with no "right" or "one size fits all" answer. In future chapters, we will address in more detail some of the positive and negative emotional impacts of a medical career as a whole. But we will start here with a discussion of those elements specifically as they pertain to medical training (med school and residency).

The physical toll of residency is considerable and may be easier to comprehend than the emotional impact, as the hours and workload are within the realm of public knowledge. People have likely seen numerous TV shows and movies which depict the lives of medical and surgical residents. Though they are not always true to real-life medical practice, these media often do focus on something which is realistic: the rigorous and hectic nature of resident life. We have already touched on the work hours, with residents frequently surpassing eighty-hour workweeks (for reference, forty hours is generally considered the standard workweek in America). There is no doubt that the workload required to complete residency (and med school rotations) can be grueling. Sleep deprivation in residency is certainly a factor. Working twelve- to fourteen-hour days on busy rotations does not leave much time for sleep when you consider eating, chores, or any leftover time for leisure. Overnight and twenty-four-hour shifts are commonplace, as residents cover the hospital day and night. I can say from personal experience that over time, this does take a physical toll on the body. But the grind does ultimately produce skill and expertise, and there can be a lot of professional satisfaction in the hard work along the way. Hopefully, residents and medical students can find enough balance throughout the process to maintain their physical (and emotional) health.

The psychological/emotional impact of residency is something else altogether and is certainly more difficult to describe and comprehend. This impact is certainly related to the physical toll of long days and sleepless nights. But there are also ups and downs felt in the heart and mind more than the body: growing from a frightened and flustered med student to an excited but anxious intern to a comfortable and seasoned resident; learning to deliver the news of a difficult diagnosis such as multiple sclerosis or an intracranial bleed which has left a patient unresponsive; weathering the storm of an abusive patient or a disgruntled family member; all the while feeling the pride of growing into a competent physician and supporting your patients with both clinical care and human compassion. I recall many of these poignant moments, two of which we experienced together in Chapter 3. These deep emotional experiences, both positive and negative, are unique to the practice of medicine. Medical school and especially residency training contain such a high concentration of these experiences due to the pace/rigor of the work as well as the rapid growth/learning that trainees undergo throughout these years. This makes residency, in my opinion, an experience as close to the proverbial emotional roller coaster as possible.

One of the toughest emotional components of residency and medical school alike is an ongoing feeling of incompetence. Due to the steep learning curve, as well as the fact that mastering clinical care requires learning a vast array of skills in different work environments, the medical student and even the intern often feel like a perpetual novice. Similar to what we covered before in our discussion of medical school rotations, even during intern year there is the constant challenge of moving to a new rotation/clinical setting each month. For example, first an internal medicine intern is on the medical wards in the hospital; next they are off to several outpatient clinics, often a different one every day or even half day; next to a specialty rotation in gastroenterology; next to the ICU; then to the cardiac ICU; then back to the hospital wards; next to a specialty clinic in nephrology; and so on and so forth. For much of the year, many if not all interns are dealing with the stress of having a new job every month and having to start fresh just as they are gaining some proficiency (let alone mastery). This component of the residency experience is emotionally challenging. To work tirelessly day in and day out and not necessarily see the tangible effects of that labor is difficult. In a typical job outside of healthcare, one might work in a single department for months or even years, building new skills sequentially, growing and becoming proficient at one task before mastering another. But in the case of the resident, the variety of clinical rotations and broad array of subspecialties make it hard to gain comfort and proficiency for at least a year or so. Interns must exercise patience, knowing that all their hard work is leading to growth, even though it may not always feel that way.

Yet through this all, the intern and resident slowly gain a broad base of knowledge and skills which build upon one another. Steadily they develop a repertoire of experiences and knowledge that make each subsequent month a little easier. The stress of these novel encounters starts to abate as experience and confidence grow. Ultimately, the resident does begin to attain mastery; in doing so, they become more and more comfortable in their role. Once experience begins to accumulate (for me this became noticeable at approximately the midpoint of my three-year residency), the work starts to become more fun. Certainly, there were fun moments throughout, even during intern year; but as I moved on to my second and third years of residency, I began to feel good at my job. I found myself feeling comfortable leading the team of med students and interns on rounds, teaching important concepts as I had been taught by my predecessors. When I received a call from the ER for a new admission with an infection in the liver, a blood clot in the lung, or a mass in the bone, I knew the appropriate workup and management to initiate. I certainly did not know it all, but I felt comfortable evaluating and treating patients, speaking with them confidently about their care. I also felt comfortable recognizing the limits of my knowledge, asking for help and seeking more answers if needed. This feeling of proficiency leads to an even more important feeling: purpose—that one belongs and has an important role to play in the healthcare system. This purpose is essential for professional satisfaction in any field in the long run. We all strive to feel that we are good at something, that we play a key role and provide some meaningful service to the world. Residency is inherently challenging because it requires a great deal of time and effort to reach that point; but by virtue of this fact, achieving proficiency and striving toward expertise during residency become even more gratifying.

On that note, residency for me was a much more positive work experience than third and fourth years of medical school. In residency, I felt I truly had that purpose and I was working each day to achieve something meaningful. Being employed (despite a relatively low salary) and providing an integral service to my patients and the function of my institution provided me loads more personal gratification than medical school did. I felt I belonged. This feeling, coupled with a growing understanding of medicine which allowed me to tangibly help people every day, made residency a positive experience in many ways. The opportunity to better your patients' lives every day is uniquely fulfilling, and residency offers that in abundance.

There is undoubtedly considerable adversity throughout residency as well. With each positive comes a counteracting negative, or so it seems. One particular challenge of residency for me and several of my colleagues was the lack of financial gratification. This was actually most pronounced in medical school, as despite countless days and nights of grueling work, we were actually paying (rather than earning) hundreds of dollars each day. This plays a hard psychological trick on a young person, though this is not totally unique to medicine. I personally did not anticipate how challenging it was to be three to four years out of undergrad, feeling that I had achieved about as highly as I possibly could to that point of my career, with nothing to show for it financially. In fact, not only did I not have any financial gain to speak of, I incurred six figures of debt. Observing my similarly bright and driven friends from undergrad who had chosen other careers enjoy the financial fruits of their labor was a stark contrast to my experience. If you pursue medicine, you must know and accept this: you are making a sacrifice, both emotional and financial. You will need to have the patience to forgo some of the pleasures many aspire to: traveling as much as you might like, buying nice gifts for your family and friends, or purchasing a home in your twenties. The majority of these things will be very difficult (though not impossible) to attain as a medical trainee, and you will need to be patient before you get them.

On a similar note, medical school and residency require sacrificing important life moments. You will likely miss out on weddings, birthdays, and life events due to a grueling work schedule in the hospital or operating room. You will work weekends and nights, sometimes for months at a time. If you have a significant other, children, close friends, or family, you will spend plenty of nights away from them caring for sick patients.

I recall several instances throughout residency when I felt this toll, some more painful than others. I missed a family reunion by the beach with my grandparents, aunts, uncles, and cousins. I missed multiple trips to visit my best friends from college who lived in another city. I missed a huge concert which would have been my first time seeing my all-time favorite musical artist. I was once called into the ICU for a thirty-hour shift only minutes after my now wife had arrived from out of town to see me. I missed family birthdays and special occasions like Thanksgiving, Christmas, and New Years. I missed all these moments because I needed to work and could not get time off during residency, time away from the hospital. I even recall that on some occasions when I was able to make events like Thanksgiving with my family, I was not truly present. The anxiety of a stressful rotation or sick patients hung over me and I could not enjoy the moment as I had I the past. This was one of the hardest realizations for me during residency. Not only was I dealing with physical absence from important moments with loved ones, but also emotional absence. The stress at times pervaded my life outside the hospital which was difficult to deal with. Luckily, with time I grew more comfortable with my skills and more capable of compartmentalizing my professional hardships. Today (for the most part) I am able to enjoy my time with loved ones independent of the stress of caring for the sick and dying. But these are the burdens of the physician and healthcare provider: we must sacrifice important life moments because, at the end of the day, our patients need us.

Hopefully you find meaning in your work, and this meaning outweighs the hardship. But there are real sacrifices—physical, emotional, and financial—that are made on the path to a career in medicine. It is best to know about them in advance so that your career decisions are well-informed. Make no mistake, though:

nothing worthwhile is achieved without hard work. Work ethic and dedication are prerequisites of success regardless of the field you choose. I can almost guarantee that another career path will not heap lavish rewards upon you in the absence of sweat and sacrifice. But as always, my purpose here is not to compare or to discourage but to educate. The premed hopeful must know what they are destined for: a years-long commitment of hard work and sacrifice with many triumphs and highs along the way. If done for the right reasons, it will all be worth it.

Part IV: Practice

Chapter 11: What is Attending Life Really Like?

Understanding the experience of a fully trained, practicing physician should be a matter of utmost importance for an aspiring premedical student. But all too often it is overlooked and not explored deeply. Students (very understandably) tend to focus on the most immediate and daunting challenge—getting into med school—at the expense of considering what life will be like once medical training is complete. It is also inherently difficult to gain the perspective and exposure needed to comprehend a career which is likely a decade away, particularly when it is shrouded by limited information and common misconceptions.

This cannot and should not be. A typical career in medicine will last thirty to forty years; if you are to spend the better part of your adult life dedicated to a pursuit, it will benefit you greatly to understand what the path will entail and what life will look like once you get there.

The various specialty options for residency training were listed before (see Chapter 10). They provide a scaffold upon which to build an understanding of the career choices available to physicians. From the outset, it is important to keep in mind two key concepts regarding career options within medicine:

1. There are numerous specialty options, and the experience and day-to-day practice of each will vary greatly. The general concepts of a career as a physician will be similar in all specialties, but the details of the job—tasks, procedures, and patient care performed—may differ significantly.

2. It is quite rare that a medical student selects a specialty to pursue and does not deviate from that to a different choice over the long course of medical education and training. Most med students change their chosen specialty at some point during medical school, sometimes multiple times. This is to be expected as there is a huge amount of learning and exposure that occurs during these formative years. Without having had the experience of medical school, how could one be totally sure of their specialty choice? Thus, it is always important to keep an open mind when planning a career in medicine.

Taken together, these two points demonstrate that there is no way to know exactly what your future career will hold or what it will look like on a day-to-day basis. But by reading the pages that follow, you will gain a better understanding of the specialty options available to you, the various settings in which physicians practice, and the general themes of the attending experience. Remember to always keep an open mind and use the knowledge gained here as another tool to help you navigate the winding path toward your future career.

Fellowship Options

Exploring each and every fellowship option within the various fields of medicine is a significant task which is again somewhat beyond the scope of our discussion. At this point in your education or consideration of a career in medicine, it is more than sufficient to be aware of the nineteen residency specialty options listed in Chapter 10. With that said, many fellowship options do exist, as almost every specialty provides the opportunity to complete further training/sub-specialization within that field. Below is a list of some of the fellowship options for each specialty. This list is not exhaustive but does include most of the fellowship options in each field of practice. It is a useful resource for understanding the more nuanced career options that lie ahead in your future medical career.

1. Anesthesiology
    a. Critical Care
    b. Cardiac Anesthesia
    c. Neurologic Anesthesia
    d. Obstetric Anesthesia
    e. Pain Medicine
    f. Pediatric Anesthesia

2. Ear, Nose, and Throat Surgery (also known as Head and Neck Surgery or Otolaryngology)
    a. Neurotology
    b. Pediatric Otolaryngology
    c. Plastics/Reconstructive Head and Neck Surgery
    d. Sleep Medicine

3. Emergency Medicine
    a. Critical Care
    b. Hyperbaric Medicine
    c. Pediatric Emergency Medicine
    d. Sports Medicine

e. Toxicology
　　f. Wilderness Medicine
4. Family Medicine
　　a. Geriatrics
　　b. Integrative Medicine
　　c. Palliative Care
　　d. Sports Medicine
　　e. Women's Health
5. General surgery
　　a. Breast surgery
　　b. Cardiothoracic surgery
　　c. Colorectal surgery
　　d. Pediatric surgery
　　e. Surgical Oncology
　　f. Transplant surgery
　　g. Vascular surgery
6. Internal Medicine
　　a. Cardiology
　　b. Endocrinology
　　c. Gastroenterology
　　d. Geriatrics
　　e. Hospital Medicine
　　f. Nephrology
　　g. Oncology
　　h. Palliative Care
　　i. Pulmonology
　　j. Rheumatology
　　k. Sleep medicine
　　l. Sports medicine
7. Neurology
　　a. Epilepsy
　　b. Headache

    c. Movement Disorders
    d. Multiple Sclerosis and Neuroimmunology
    e. Neurocritical Care
    f. Neuromuscular Diseases
    g. Vascular Neurology
8. Neurosurgery
    a. Advanced Endoscopic & Open Skull Base Surgery
    b. Epilepsy Surgery
    c. Neurosurgical Oncology
    d. Radiosurgery
    e. Spine Surgery
    f. Stereotactic & Functional Neurosurgery
9. Obstetrics/Gynecology
    a. Complex Family Planning
    b. Female Pelvic Medicine and Reconstructive Surgery
    c. Gynecologic Oncology
    d. Maternal-fetal Medicine
    e. Reproductive Endocrinology and Infertility
10. Ophthalmology
    a. Cornea & External Disease
    b. Glaucoma
    c. Neuro-Ophthalmology
    d. Ophthalmic Plastic & Reconstructive Surgery
    e. Pediatric & Strabismus
    f. Vitreoretinal Surgery
    g. Uveitis & Medical Retina
11. Orthopedic Surgery
    a. Adult Reconstruction and Arthroplasty
    b. Foot and Ankle Surgery
    c. Hand Surgery
    d. Pediatrics
    e. Sports
    f. Trauma

12. Pathology
    a. Cytopathology
    b. Dermatopathology
    c. Hematopathology
    d. Medical Microbiology
    e. Molecular Genetic Pathology
    f. Neuropathology
    g. Surgical Pathology
    h. Transfusion Medicine
13. Pediatrics
    a. Cardiology
    b. Endocrinology
    c. Gastroenterology
    d. Nephrology
    e. Neurology
    f. Oncology
    g. Palliative Care
    h. Pulmonology
    i. Rheumatology
14. Physical Medicine and Rehabilitation
    a. Brain Injury
    b. Pediatric Rehabilitation
    c. Spinal Cord Injury
    d. Sports Medicine
15. Psychiatry
    a. Addiction Medicine
    b. Child and Adolescent Psychiatry
    c. Forensic Psychiatry
    d. Geriatric Psychiatry
    e. Interventional Psychiatry
    f. Neuropsychiatry
    g. Sleep Medicine

16. Radiation Oncology
    a. Advanced Radiation Oncology
    b. Brachytherapy
    c. Proton Therapy
17. Radiology
    a. Breast Imaging
    b. Cardiothoracic Imaging
    c. Cross-Sectional Body Imaging
    d. Interventional Radiology
    e. Interventional Neuroradiology
    f. Musculoskeletal Imaging
    g. Neuroradiology
    h. Nuclear Medicine
18. Urology
    a. Endourology and Stone Disease
    b. Female Pelvic Medicine and Reconstructive Surgery
    c. Men's Health
    d. Minimally Invasive Surgery
    e. Prosthetics and Genitourinary Reconstruction
    f. Urologic Oncology

With the extensive list provided here, you have a snapshot of nearly all the specialty options available to you in a career as a physician. There is a great breadth (even a cornucopia) of areas in which to practice medicine. Again, do not sweat the nuances of this list as they are not necessary to know in detail. The big picture is what matters. Even for myself, as a practicing hospitalist who deals with many of these specialties daily, there are several fellowships listed above that I was not previously familiar with. Furthermore, avoid becoming prematurely preoccupied with what specialty is best for you, as odds are your priorities and preferences will change over time. Keep with you the general idea/concept of this list—the knowledge that several specialties/fellowships exist to choose from down the line. This concept is a great insight into the depth of opportunity in medicine, which will ultimately help you navigate its complex landscape.

An important idea to note is that it is not imperative that any graduating resident complete a fellowship. There are countless physicians out there doing great work in family medicine, general internal medicine, general pediatrics, general surgery, psychiatry, neurology, radiology, and more who did not pursue fellowship. There is no expectation that a premed student should aspire to the most sub-specialized training. If one of these fellowship pathways fits your interests and personal goals, that is great. But if not, that is also perfectly okay. Remember that college, medical school, and residency are quite enough education and training. They comprise a long and challenging road that produces well-trained physicians. Those physicians who have not completed fellowship are just as crucial to the healthcare system as those who have. Without each of these important physician specialties, the system would not function. Ultimately, wherever your intellectual interests lie is the best path to pursue your future career.

Practice Settings

Once you have grasped the broad array of subspecialties within medicine, it is perhaps more important to learn about the different settings and practice types through which medical care is delivered. Your experience will differ significantly based on which setting you choose to practice in. This is a key concept to understand; it is one that would otherwise be difficult to discern as a premed student without direct clinical experience in healthcare.

The first major distinction drawn between practice settings in medicine is between "academics" and "non-academics." Let's define these terms (or at least what they typically describe) to provide a better understanding of the two main options available in clinical medicine.

Academic Medicine

Academics refers to the practice of medicine at a university medical center which typically has one or all of the following components: a medical school, a residency program, and ongoing medical research within the undergraduate/medical school campuses. An academic physician is one who practices at hospitals/clinics which are affiliated with a university and the above components, such as Massachusetts General Hospital which is associated with Harvard or Ronald Reagan Medical Center which is associated with UCLA. These physicians can technically practice both independently or in conjunction with trainees, but typically at least some (and sometimes all) of the academic physician's clinical practice will be spent supervising residents and med students. Thus, the clinical experience of the academic physician is very different from that of the independent physician working in a non-academic setting in the community (more on that in a moment).

In the inpatient setting, an academic attending physician is the head of a large team of medical students and residents who are tasked with caring for a group of patients admitted to the hospital. Much of the direct patient care (such as orders, procedures, notes, etc.) is completed by the students and residents as part of their medical training, as discussed in previous chapters. The job of the attending is to oversee the whole group, ensuring appropriate patient care is being delivered while providing guidance, feedback, and education. This last component is a large difference which exists between academic and non-academic medicine: an academic attending will often be expected to teach medical students and residents daily. For many, this is a draw of academic medicine, as they enjoy passing knowledge on to the next generation of physicians. For others, it is a deterrent, as they would rather focus on direct patient care and avoid the challenges that can come with teaching.

In the outpatient setting, academic physicians will run their own clinics, with some portion of their day being spent precepting/educating medical students and residents. Again, the attending will be charged with overseeing patient care to ensure appropriate decisions are being made, while also teaching key points to trainees along the way.

Another important component of practicing in an academic setting is performing medical research. Academic attendings will do this to varying degrees; some spend a majority of their time on research, running a lab and multiple research studies. It is not uncommon for research-oriented physicians to spend eighty percent of their time on research and only twenty percent on clinical work (they are hired in this capacity). Some MDs may even elect to pursue research full-time, though this occurs in a minority of cases and is more common among MD-PhDs. Other physicians practice almost completely clinically, with a small component of their work spent on research and/or formal education of medical students and residents. Though it can take many forms, most academic physicians will need to perform at least some sort of scholarly pursuit (either research or formal teaching) to maintain their academic appointment and progress toward promotions.

Finally, it is important to note that the pay in academic medicine tends to be lower than in private practice (though there can certainly be exceptions to this trend). According to a 2016 survey of 35,000 physicians, academic physicians made an average of thirteen percent less than non-academic physicians in the same field[1]. There is also considerable variability in this pay gap based on specialty; cardiologists, for example, made fifty-two percent less in the academic setting than non-academics, according to the same survey[1]. Though certainly not the bottom line for happiness and satisfaction during a career in medicine, finances are a consideration when comparing academic and non-academic practice settings.

Non-Academic Medicine

Medical practice outside of the academic setting can vary greatly, but I will group these practice settings together and describe them here, as academic versus non-academic medicine is the most important distinction for a student or young physician-in-training to understand. Non-academic medicine, as the name implies, is medicine practiced in a setting not associated with a university, medical school, or residency program. It therefore places the physician in a more independent role, in which they directly provide the medical care to the patient rather than overseeing a team of trainees. Thus, teaching is a far smaller component of non-academic medicine, with the exception of education given to other providers such as nurses or physician peers (and of course the daily education all physicians provide to their patients). In some circumstances, providers such as nurse practitioners and physician's assistants also work alongside non-academic physicians, providing patient care under the attending's supervision. Incidentally, these "mid-level" providers can also practice in academic settings but tend to be less common there, as medical students and residents perform much of the patient care.

Within non-academic medicine, two main types of practice exist. The most well-known is private practice, or medical care delivered in a practice completely owned by physicians and not by a hospital, medical group, or health system. This is the prototype of the physician who is his or her own boss, running a business which provides care to a panel of patients who choose to see that doctor. Private practices vary in size, ranging from individual practices to groups owned jointly by several physicians. The second major non-academic practice setting is medical groups which are owned by a hospital or health system. Examples include Kaiser Permanente in California, Christus Health in Texas, or Cleveland Clinic in the Midwest. These often-sizable entities and others like them employ large numbers of physicians in a group medical practice, typically with several different specialties. They can be localized to a particular region, such as my own medical system (Sharp Healthcare) located in San Diego, California; or they can be more geographically widespread, such as Kaiser Permanente, which is located in several states across the country. These systems are not owned by the physicians themselves, and thus differ fundamentally from private practice. The physician is an employee rather than an owner/operator of the business. Depending on an individual's preferences, this may be a pro or a con. Private practice carries the significant responsibility of operating a business, from obtaining the physical space, to employing the support staff, to running the billing/financials. But along with those responsibilities come more autonomy and often greater financial upside. Meanwhile, financial opportunity may be more limited as an employee in a large medical group, but this setting provides freedom from the responsibility and challenges of running and operating the business.

So how many physicians work in private practice? In the 2020 Physician Practice Benchmark Survey conducted by the AMA, forty-nine percent of physicians worked in practices completely owned by physicians, down from fifty-four percent in 2018 (and sixty percent in 2012)[2]. A caveat to this, which I can attest to from personal and peer experience in California and elsewhere, is that in larger cities/markets it is becoming increasingly more difficult and therefore less common to work in private practice. In many populous cities, large medical groups/entities like those already mentioned have a stronghold on the healthcare market share and continue to grow each year. In other words, large medical groups are gaining more patients and hospital contracts over time as they have the ability to provide more services by one centralized organization; thus, true private practices are slowly being phased out in many large metropolitan areas. In smaller and less populated areas of the country, private practice remains more common and more feasible.

Ultimately, each setting (academics, private practice, or large medical group practice) has unique features as well as pros and cons. It is not necessarily crucial early in one's educational career to know which setting they prefer; but it does help to understand the variable experiences and the different opportunities available in each setting as an attending. As med students and residents grow and mature throughout training, they gravitate toward whatever setting is best suited to their priorities. By knowing early on that these different settings exist and have unique features, your understanding of the landscape of medicine is far more complete. You are ahead of the game.

Alternative Career Options for Physicians (Non-Clinical Work)

While there are many alternatives to a career in medicine—ranging from engineering to the arts, biotech to law, finance to journalism—there are also multiple alternative, non-clinical options available to physicians after completing medical education or training. Some find that their talents and interests have a better application than patient care. Others find happiness in diversifying their pursuits, continuing patient care while taking on non-clinical roles as well. Let's explore some of these options to understand how else physicians can apply their knowledge and training.

The most obvious example of diversification of career options within medicine is medical research. In some ways, this is part and parcel of a career in medicine, as most physicians complete at least some research over the course of their medical education and training. Therefore, I will not describe this in great detail here. Most everyone is aware that a physician can always make research, either clinical or basic science, a significant portion of their career.

Another career option that becomes available to physicians, often over the course of time and with years of experience, is medical administration and leadership. All large entities such as hospitals and medical groups need structured leadership systems to oversee and operate themselves, perform administrative duties, and ensure that things run effectively. Physicians in these leadership roles might be responsible for hiring/recruiting new doctors, evaluating finances and productivity, mediating disputes, and creating systems/protocols for patient care. Physicians can pursue such leadership positions throughout their career. Some choose to gain formal education and training, such as an MBA, to bolster their skills in business and administration. Others learn on the job through years of work in hospitals, clinics, and other healthcare organizations. If one has a mind for such things, coupled with interpersonal and diplomatic skills, they can go far as a leader and administrator in the healthcare world.

Other physicians have interests in healthcare policy or disciplines such epidemiology. Typically, those with such interests pursue higher education beyond their MD degree, such as an MPH or other Master's degrees like epidemiology or clinical research (recall Chapter 6). These additional degrees are tools in the arsenal of a physician's knowledge base; they can act as stepping-stones to other career options, such as development of healthcare policy for a physician with an MPH, for example.

One particularly intriguing career option for MDs, which premed students may not recognize, is the opportunity to move into industry. This means using medical knowledge and training to work in business, outside the actual practice of medicine. Some physicians become entrepreneurs, starting their own companies and developing their own products. Others use their expertise to become consultants or medical advisors to healthcare or technology companies. Be aware that this is certainly a minority of physicians, but this route is a viable career option after med school or residency training for those interested. I would personally never recommend becoming a physician in order to pursue a career in industry, as to me the opportunity cost of time and money lost during education and training is too great for the potential reward at the finish line. If your interests clearly lie more strongly in business, economics, engineering, or technology, it is likely more efficient to pursue that directly rather than through medical training. With that said, it is good to be aware that some physicians do shift gears later and apply their training to business pursuits rather than the practice of medicine. If these interests arise after pursuing medical education, industry can certainly be a very exciting and fruitful career option for a physician.

Ultimately, knowing all the options and paths available to physicians after completing training provides you the most comprehensive view of the field you are choosing. It's a broad and varied world out there in medicine. Variety is the spice of life, and there is certainly a plethora of spices to tantalize the palate of the trained physician.

Now that we have considered each step on the road to becoming a physician—premed, med school, residency, fellowship, and attending life—it is time to take a nuanced look at the factors which will affect your experience once you get there. As aspiring physicians, we often view the completion of training as the finish line, a symbolic representation of the end of an epic journey. But this, in fact, is not the reality. Completing medical training and moving on to a career as an attending is only the next step in a physician's professional journey. We should view it as a continuum of experience; once you reach that point, you will find a new set of successes and challenges. You will still work hard as an attending, of course, and will need to navigate complex decisions to find the right personal and professional balance. As we take a look at some key factors, think back to your personal goals and values, which we have touched on prior. Consider what is most important to you, as this will help you lay a solid mental foundation for your future goals.

The first factor we will consider, one which is hard to escape when considering any career, is money. Let's take a detailed look at the key financial implications of a career in medicine, and what that will mean for the life of a physician.

Chapter 12: Financial Implications of a Career as a Physician

"Doctors are rich."
"I want to become a doctor and make lots of money."
"They're doctors...they must be wealthy, right?"

These notions regarding the financial rewards of the medical profession are not uncommon in the minds of the general public. To truly understand the financial implications of a career as a physician though, one must first consider something quite simple, but perhaps shocking: these ideas are to some degree based on a modern misconception. The financial experience of a physician is typically much more complex; it is not necessarily a fast and easy route to financial success, a means of rapidly accumulating wealth. Physicians certainly earn high salaries, and there are significant financial benefits to a career in medicine. The profession makes for a good living which is enough to provide a comfortable (and sometimes even luxurious) life. It would be wrong to deny that. But as we touched on in Chapter 4, a career as a physician carries considerable financial challenges which accompany those benefits: the massive rise in the cost of medical education has led to significant physician debt[1]; low income during long residency training delays the physician's earning potential; and physician salaries have not always risen at a rate commensurate with other industries[2] or even inflation[3]. For these reasons and others, money in and of itself is never the right reason to choose a career in medicine. But it is important for prospective doctors to understand what can be expected financially during their future career. Let's explore in greater detail the existing reality of finances in the medical profession and how this may affect your future as a physician.

Debt

First and foremost, the aspiring premedical student needs to understand the amount of debt associated with medical education. Simply put, medical school is extremely expensive[4]. There are a select few individuals who are able to avoid using loans to fund medical school: those with significant prior earning/savings, typically from a previous career in another line of work; students with parents/families who are financially equipped to fund their medical school tuition; very few students who earn a substantial scholarship; or those who have committed to either an MD-PhD program or the armed forces and therefore receive medical education at low or no cost. These individuals are to be congratulated as they have bypassed one of the most challenging aspects of medical training: debt. The majority of the medical student population, though, will need to take out loans (federal, subsidized, or private) to fund the substantial cost of med school tuition as well as room, board, and other life expenses.

According to recent data published by the AAMC, the median cost of medical school tuition (not including housing or living expenses) in 2022-2023 was the following: $41,095 for public in-state; $65,744 for public out-of-state; $67,294 for private in-state; and $67,855 for private out-of-state[4]. Overall, the average cost of medical school is $57,574 per year and $218,792 total over the course of four years[5]. The financial burden of medical school is substantial and can be significantly higher than that of undergrad, depending on the institution you attended. Consequently, by virtue of sheer mathematical inevitability, the average graduating med student finishes school with a large amount of debt. According to the AAMC, seventy-three percent of medical students graduate with some debt and the median debt was exactly $200,000 in 2019[6].

Let me take a moment to pause here. This number may be difficult to comprehend for the average undergrad (or even high school) student reading this text early on their path to a career in medicine. I will try not to belabor it too much, as cost is not the most important factor when considering a degree and it is simply an unavoidable component of medical training. But I do think it is important to at least recognize that $200,000 or more of debt (and much more for some—remember the above number is only the median) is a huge number which will typically take several years to pay off. Depending on what part of the country one resides in, $200,000 could be the cost of a condo or even a freestanding home. A home is often considered the largest, and therefore most consequential, purchase of one's life. Medical school can pose a comparable cost, or at least one in the same ballpark. But it is typically not viewed in this way, as such a significant financial undertaking. Students should at least be aware of this factor and recognize the financial burden which they incur when choosing to go to medical school. It is far from insignificant.

I discuss this concept not to deter or incite fear. Rather, my purpose is to inform and thereby empower premed students. It is important to understand that choosing medical school (as well as other health professional or graduate schools) is a significant financial decision, which you will almost certainly have to fund after your education. This can take years, and one should be prepared for that process when making the initial decision.

In medicine, there is the added complexity of at least a few and possibly several years of residency training which are accompanied by a relatively low salary when compared to the level of skill and education the job entails. Again, consider the notion that doctors are very wealthy. Residency salaries are relatively standardized nationwide such that most residents begin their intern year making between $55,00 and $65,000 per year with the current median being $60,942[7]. (Note that this is an increase compared to my era when the range was closer to $45,000 to $55,000 per year; so there is some sequential improvement in resident salaries with inflation). The annual salary increases by a small percentage each year of residency/fellowship, such that an eighth-year resident or fellow is usually making a base salary of approximately $82,000 on average, based on the most recent data from the AAMC[7]. Now this is certainly enough to pay the bills and even care for one's family. I certainly would not scoff at this amount of money. But the sum becomes increasingly inadequate when one considers that residents and even fellows routinely work eighty or more hours per week, essentially double the average American workweek. The salary simply does not match the hours worked, nor does it reflect the level of expertise gained and the service rendered. These are full-fledged physicians working long hours, weekends, and nights caring for real, live patients. They possess years of experience delivering medical care to those in need. These physicians are essentially the lifeblood of academic hospitals and medical systems, providing a huge amount of the day-to-day medical care. The take-home point is that the residency salary is not huge, and it becomes smaller in light of the effort it requires to both reach and complete residency. When you consider that, and the earning potential of other jobs with consummate levels of education and expertise, the realization is that residents are not in a particularly robust financial position. To make matters worse, the majority of these residents have six figures of debt (as noted before) and are often unable to make a significant dent in that debt until after residency due to their limited salary. Consequently, trainees incur a growing amount of interest on already considerable loan principals; they are often saddled with their debt for at least a decade or more before they have the true financial capability to pay it back. Therein lies the first financial challenge of a career in medicine: due to debt incurred by education and a relatively low salary as a resident and fellow, medical trainees will have to live somewhat frugally for around a decade or more before they begin to reap the financial rewards of being an attending physician. Again, the compensation of a resident is adequate to provide for a decent life. But by no means are physicians wealthy early in their careers. This should not be a deterrent for aspiring students, but a valuable nugget of information which makes them better prepared when approaching a medical career. The cost of medical education is simply an unavoidable truth which must be recognized.

Opportunity Cost

The second key point that future physicians must understand is opportunity cost. Though this is an economic concept, it is very relevant to a career in medicine (and likewise to long education/training in other fields of work; incidentally it is a powerful transactional concept which I think has relevance to many life decisions). Opportunity cost is defined as "the loss of potential gain from other alternatives when one alternative is chosen." It essentially identifies the cost of choosing one path when multiple paths are available, as the path(s) not chosen may have some potential gain or benefit which was lost by opting for the alternative. This concept can be applied to many instances in life when we encounter a crossroad, a branchpoint providing multiple options with different outcomes. Opportunity cost is especially pertinent to the decision to attend graduate school and bears no greater relevance to any field than medicine.

The primary opportunity cost of choosing a career as a physician is the loss of potential earnings if one were to choose another path. Because it requires the longest training of any professional/advanced degree, a career as a medical doctor carries the greatest opportunity cost. With four years of med school providing no earning, followed by anywhere from three to eight years of residency/fellowship providing lower salaries than could likely be achieved elsewhere, the opportunity cost of medical training is significant (some might say immense). But let's acknowledge that the concept of significant opportunity cost associated with the residency and fellowship years does rely on the notion that an individual would have higher earning potential in an alternative field. While this is not a guarantee, let me describe why it is a reasonable assumption in many cases.

First and foremost, all premed students who are accepted and matriculate to a medical school program have at least a college degree. Suffice it to say that these individuals are highly functioning, as they needed to have high GPA's, good test scores, significant clinical and research experience, and more in order to get accepted to medical school. By and large, this a group of relatively intelligent and hard-working individuals. It is not a significant stretch to assume that these skills would likely translate to success in other fields as well. Now I am not saying that a med student or a physician could perform any job and I mean no disrespect to the expertise and merit of any other profession. Rather, I am suggesting that med students have attributes, most importantly hard work and diligence, which would likely help them achieve success in other fields if they were to choose one. I also believe this would be true of many college graduates pursuing higher education in other disciplines besides medicine.

Next, consider that at the point when a medical student would graduate and finally begin earning a salary in residency, an analogous individual in the workforce would already have at least four years of work experience under their belt. Those four years of work would provide the non-medical individual time for professional growth and potentially promotion. Thus, it is very reasonable to propose that a highly functioning individual four-plus years out of college working in industry or other spheres would have an earning potential higher than the average starting resident salary of approximately $60,000. And therein lies the opportunity cost of the post-medical-school years: the potential earnings lost while a resident/fellow trains for years and slowly ascends toward the attending salary. Though not as easily visible as the debt incurred from medical education, this opportunity cost is still important to consider, as residency training can stretch for many years before the physician reaches their full earning potential.

To drive this point home, let us take for example two hard-working, intelligent friends exiting college, one to pursue med school and the other to pursue a career as an engineer in the tech industry. The latter can certainly be a very lucrative path; but more important than earning potential is earning duration: the engineer graduate heading off to work for Google or Instagram will start earning immediately and begin building their net worth right away. With hard work and some good decision making, in a few years they may have the privilege of buying a new home or reaching other financial milestones.

Meanwhile, the med student will start an equally exciting process of rapid and intense learning in medical school. But this individual will work hard as a med student for a minimum of four years, not earning money but rather amassing considerable debt despite tremendous effort. Their earning will be delayed by at least four years until they complete med school. The majority of the time, they will start their earning career with tens or hundreds of thousands of dollars of debt, as we have discussed. This is not by any fault of theirs, but simply is a reality of medical education.

The med student will have to delay gratification and may watch their friend reach important financial milestones much sooner. They will have to exercise patience and restraint, living more frugally than they might have otherwise. This opportunity cost of medical training is important to understand; it requires waiting four years to earn money, followed by a relatively low earning potential in residency compared to the years of training and expertise that a resident possesses. It requires sacrifice and it will likely have some impact on your quality of life during this time.

The Promised Land

Now that I have painted this realistic (yet somewhat bleak) picture of the financial outlook of medical education/training, let's consider the flip side, which is quite positive. Once a resident or fellow completes training and moves on to become an attending physician, the game completely changes. In 2023, the average physician salary was $260,000 for a primary care physician and $339,000 for a specialist[8]. This number is difficult to interpret in that it is an average of dozens of disparate entities, as each medical subspecialty and geographical region has a different earning potential. But what it does represent is that the practicing physician is essentially guaranteed a very solid salary, one which is adequate for living a comfortable or perhaps even affluent life. Choosing medicine provides a "high financial floor," or in other words a high guaranteed salary. Though it also has a relatively "low ceiling," which we will touch upon later, there is no denying that medicine eventually provides a high guaranteed salary which a physician can bank on. If you seek a clear path to a salary which is typically $200,000 or beyond, medicine will provide that opportunity and eventual stability. Bear in mind that the destination comes by way of about a decade of financial hurdles which we discussed prior. But ultimately, a physician who completes their training pathway is essentially assured a good (and potentially great) salary. This is undoubtedly one of the biggest strengths of a career in medicine.

Another positive financial aspect of life as a physician is less volatility and increased job security when compared to other industries. Healthcare jobs are typically more stable than, say, a position at a tech start-up or a job in the financial industry. Medical systems are not immune to hard times and even failures; therefore, it is not impossible for a physician or healthcare professional to be laid off as in other industries. Yet, in general, this is less common in medicine because healthcare at its core will always be necessary; in fact, it is typically increasing in demand, as our population is living longer with greater medical complexity and need for medical care. Medicine is never going out of business. Certainly, there are financial challenges for private practices, hospitals, and large medical groups alike; but a physician's skillset is very likely to remain in demand, providing a degree of job security which is not present in all industries.

When thinking in greater detail about the financial outlook of a career as a practicing physician, there is both significant upside and considerable limitation. Though this two-sided nature may seem paradoxical, we have already touched on some of the reasons why this is true (debt and opportunity cost versus high guaranteed salary). But there is even more to the story. Let's illustrate this concept.

The highest earning medical specialties such as cardiology, orthopedic surgery, or neurosurgery have high salaries which can easily top $500,000 and sometimes approach $1,000,000 depending on the location, setting of practice, and other factors. For example, the three aforementioned specialties had the following median salaries in 2023, as reported by Salary.com: $459,000 for interventional cardiology[9]; $525,000 for orthopedic surgery[10]; $657,000 for neurosurgery[11]. Keep in mind that these are medians with fairly large standard deviations, meaning the upper end of the spectrum is considerably higher.

Those salaries are impressive and certainly nothing to scoff at. But while the floor is high and the financial potential of a career in medicine is considerable, the ceiling is still relatively low. Now this depends upon what your comparator is and what you consider a truly high salary. When I argue that medicine has a low ceiling, this is in comparison to the earning potential at the peak of other fields such as business, technology, or finance, which can be considerably higher. To further examine this point, take the following example into consideration.

At a highly regarded academic institution where I have experience and ongoing contact, the highest physician earner made slightly over $1.7 million in 2021. This is openly published information[12] which is offered to the public online, as it is a state institution. This individual is the chief of their department in one of the highest earning, procedurally oriented specialties. Upon hearing this information, one might say "Wow, over a million dollars! That is amazing!" In many ways it is. No one needs more than a million dollars in annual salary to comfortably care for themselves and their loved ones. In fact, with such a salary one could live a decadent lifestyle, enjoying many of the finer things the world has to offer.

Now let's consider what one can earn when reaching the pinnacle of earning in a field such as technology or finance. Though these numbers can vary vastly based upon the individual circumstance, we know that the earning potential in these spheres can be far higher than one to two million dollars per year. The common thread in these alternative fields is that if someone starts their own business, hedge fund, or start-up, or reaches the highest C-suite position of a profitable company, their earning potential is much higher than a million dollars. It is not uncommon to hear of the young, bright software engineer who sold their tech start-up for eight figures (>$10,000,000) or more. Similarly, we can all think of examples of CEOs in various industries who make tens or even hundreds of millions of dollars per year[13]. Make no mistake that these individuals are the cream of the crop, literally one in a million or more in terms of aptitude, achievement, and even good fortune. Their experiences do not necessarily translate for the average individual.

But for the sake of the example, I would argue that these individuals are analogous to our top physician earner making around $1-2 million. They are the highest achievers in their respective fields, which are all of considerable importance to society. Yet the payout for each is vastly different. A million-dollar salary is far below the financial pinnacle in many fields outside of medicine. Keep in mind though, that if the physician delves into business or tech, they too can increase their earning potential, reaping the benefits of a free market which will recognize their contributions with a commensurate financial reward (i.e. capitalism). Some physicians certainly do this; but in order to exceed that million-dollar "ceiling," a physician will have to branch outside of clinical care or even medical administration into business, innovation, and entrepreneurship.

I provide this example to demonstrate a point: that a career as physician should not be considered a road to an extravagantly rich life. Spoiler alert: there is actually no guaranteed road to such a life. If there were, wouldn't many folks already be on it or at least striving to find directions to that path? Medicine certainly is a career which provides a secure financial future, allowing the physician to care for their loved ones, enjoy some luxuries, and craft their life the way they see fit. In my opinion, this is more than enough. Yet ultimately it is my duty to provide a complete account of a financial life in medicine: it has both benefits and challenges which make for a more complex reality than a simple assumption that a career as a physician will lead to surefire wealth.

Medical Malpractice Lawsuits

I will not spend a great deal of time on this topic here, as we will cover it in more detail in Chapter 13. In brief, medical malpractice is defined as[14] "any act or omission by a physician during treatment of a patient that deviates from accepted norms of practice in the medical community and causes an injury to the patient." Patients can sue physicians with the allegation that such an error occurred. I mention this now to help the reader understand that legal liability within medicine does exist and can play a role in a physician's career as well as their financial experience. Self-reported data from physician surveys demonstrate that about one third of all physicians will be sued at some point in their career[15]. Therefore, physicians need to be prepared for this possibility at any time. A consequence of medical malpractice suits is that physicians must have malpractice insurance, which of course has an associated cost. Physicians in individual or private practice will have to provide their own malpractice insurance, while most physicians in a large group practice will have it provided by their employer.

The possibility of being sued and paying a financial penalty does indeed exist and all physicians need to be cognizant of this.

But with sensible, evidence-based, conscientious practice, the chance of a lawsuit is quite low on a day-to-day or even a year-to-year basis. Furthermore, medical malpractice insurance will shoulder part of the financial burden should a lawsuit come to pass. Physicians will not face this challenge alone. As with any other form of insurance, payment upfront (by the individual or employer) for coverage will financially protect the physician down the line in the event of legal misfortune. Thus, medical malpractice typically does not affect the daily experience of the majority of physicians from either a functional or financial standpoint. Though we all must be aware and take measures to avoid them, medical malpractice lawsuits will hopefully be a small (or with any luck, nonexistent) portion of a career as a physician.

Concluding Thoughts

Discussion of finances can often be taboo when it comes to a career in medicine. I appreciate the simplest reasoning behind this notion: no one should choose medicine for money. In healthcare, we value altruism and a desire to help others above all else. I am in full agreement with these ideas, but I also feel that understanding medicine in its entirety increases the likelihood of personal fulfillment in a future career as a physician. Ignoring the financial implications altogether would be naïve and somewhat nearsighted, robbing us of the most comprehensive view of this complex career.

I would encourage any individual considering their future profession to focus on the career itself and how that pursuit matches their interests and passions, their likes and dislikes. Money should never be the primary deciding factor. But it is okay (and perhaps prudent) to consider finances as a secondary or tertiary component of the decision. With an accurate understanding of the financial aspects of the physician experience, there will be far less surprises along the way. This is a recipe for a sound career choice with the foundation necessary to provide lasting fulfillment.

Chapter 13: Common Challenges of a Career as a Physician

We have covered a great deal thus far and have already built a strong foundation of knowledge on which to launch your future career. We have discussed many positives of a medical career—from intellectual stimulation to interpersonal connection, from personal fulfillment to financial gratification. But there is still more to explore! Part of our discussion, however unpleasant, are the negative aspects of this noble pursuit.

Have you ever revealed to someone your interest in medicine, only to be met with a lukewarm, unenthusiastic, or even flat-out negative retort? Have you ever spoken to a practicing physician about your desire to join their ranks and received an exasperated sigh rather than a smile of approval? Have you ever asked a seasoned doctor if they would do it all again, and encountered more doubt than affirmation?

Unfortunately, these are not uncommon experiences for premed students and are certainly situations I remember encountering as an undergrad. Many doctors were enthusiastic and encouraging, but some were the opposite. Such is life, as there is a spectrum to each population and each experience. Some might wonder though, is there any validity to the idea that many doctors would not recommend that others pursue the same path? Perhaps yes, and perhaps no. Ultimately this is an intensely personal question for each individual physician, as the career is a great fit for some and a less-than-perfect fit for others. Regardless, the career is challenging and demanding for all those who choose it. Data do suggest that many physicians would not recommend the career to others, though I suspect this may be true for other rigorous and demanding careers as well. According to The Future of Healthcare Survey conducted in 2012 and 2018, with over 3000 physicians responding to each, the majority of doctors would not recommend healthcare as a profession to their children or family members[1,2].

This is a telling statistic; but again, it speaks to the inherent demands that a career in medicine poses. It does not paint the whole picture of the physician experience, as certainly there are plenty of positive components of the career and many doctors who are personally and professionally satisfied. But let's be a bit more thoughtful, a bit more analytical. What are the reasons some doctors are unsatisfied and unenthusiastic about encouraging the next generation? By understanding these reasons, you will be a better-informed candidate for the path that lies ahead.

Some of the answers to this question are things we have already covered in this book. Inherent to a career as a physician are the several years of intense education and clinical training. Thereafter, the job does not necessarily become easier. The practice of medicine for many physicians can continue to be physically and mentally taxing due to the sheer demands of time, effort, and daily excellence it requires.

Next is the financial aspect; as we covered in detail in Chapter 12, a career as a physician comes with significant financial hurdles (i.e. debt and opportunity cost) which must be cleared before the rewards are reaped. As we discussed, the practice of medicine is a respectable and adequate living; but for some, this is not enough. For those individuals without an understanding of the potential financial challenges, or those who may have expected to be very wealthy from their career as a physician, the financial realities of life within healthcare may be a rude awakening. I would say for most this is not true, as many of us are able to carve out a comfortable financial life coupled with satisfaction from doing meaningful work. But for some, dissatisfaction and discontent may brew from being overworked and "underpaid" (according to their own perceptions, even if underpaid is not the complete reality).

So what are the other factors which we have not yet covered that can be negative aspects of a career in medicine? Let's discuss a few in detail.

Health Risks

The risk of personal exposure to medical disease in my experience has not been on the forefront of most physicians' minds—that is, until the COVID-19 pandemic. Never before have we seen so clearly the risks that can be associated with any profession in the healthcare field, from nurses to respiratory therapists to pharmacists to physicians. With this new disease affecting our healthcare system like nothing before in the modern era, the risk of exposure to illness appears to be at an all-time high. Though this risk may be transient, as we all hope for containment of the pandemic eventually, it does highlight the unpredictable nature of a career in medicine.

But let me be clear—I have worked on the frontlines of the COVID pandemic alongside countless brave healthcare workers and have communicated with countless colleagues across the nation: not a single individual I know—doctor, nurse, or otherwise—has shirked their responsibility out of fear or hesitation. On the contrary, almost everyone I know in healthcare has stepped up, seeing this as an opportunity to give back to their community, to apply years of training to help those in need. Make no mistake, this is an honor and we do it proudly. You will as well, through whatever challenges that arise, if and when you enter the medical profession.

With that said, we must acknowledge that there is risk associated with the responsibility of being a physician. The career is both a privilege and a burden. Sadly, healthcare workers have died after contracting COVID-19 as a result of their work on the front lines. Though COVID is the prototype and perfect modern example, health risk and medical uncertainty have also been associated with other epidemics of the past: HIV in the 1980's and 1990's, previous SARS viruses in the early 2000's, the ebola virus, and other communicable diseases. The risk to healthcare workers exists primarily in the realm of infectious diseases, as direct contact with patients increases the risk of transmission.

Another example of a health risk to medical providers is exposure to bodily fluids which can also transmit a communicable disease. The medical profession makes painstaking efforts to avoid this risk, and thus it is quite rare. But occasionally mistakes do happen. For example, a healthcare worker can be accidentally stuck by a needle which was used on a patient with a transmissible disease such as hepatitis or HIV. The risk of transmission of these diseases even in the event of a needle stick is quite low, and there are treatments for these scenarios. But it is important to be aware that these small risks do exist.

Finally, fields which require physicians to be exposed to radiation (radiology, interventional radiology, cardiology, and some surgical specialties) also pose a risk. Over time, cumulative radiation does increase the risk of cancers and even some other diagnoses such as coronary artery disease. With that said, all of these specialties have protocols in place to protect physicians and mitigate this exposure, keeping the risk relatively low.

Ultimately, it is very unlikely that health risks will be a significant factor in your decision-making regarding a career in medicine. If you have a passion for medical practice and it fits your future goals, you should pursue it. Nonetheless, this risk is something to be aware of. If you choose to become a physician or other healthcare professional, these risks will be present in the background throughout your career, and you will work through them as best you can in accordance with medical guidelines. Like those that have come before you, you will navigate these challenges for the betterment of your patients and your community.

Medical Malpractice Lawsuits

Medical malpractice might carry a bit more weight when considering a career as a physician. We touched on this topic in Chapter 12, but we will consider it in a bit more detail here. Medical malpractice lawsuits are suits brought against physicians by patients with the contention that a medical error was made by the physician, causing injury or harm to the patient. This is an unfortunate but real risk to any practicing physician. It is something all of us are cognizant of to some degree throughout our medical careers.

The annual risk of malpractice lawsuits is relatively low, but over the course of a career a considerable portion of physicians will be sued for medical malpractice at some point. According to a study published by the AMA in 2016 which surveyed 3500 practicing physicians, thirty-four percent of all physicians have been sued for malpractice during their career[3]. Of course, the risk of error and liability can be mitigated if a physician stringently practices the standard of care; but most of us do practice as expected and required, and even then, mistakes occur. Neither physicians nor medical science are perfect. Furthermore, lawsuits can be brought upon physicians even when a true error did not occur, as frivolous suits unfortunately do exist. Such is the reality of litigation and liability that we must live with as physicians.

Certain specialties are at higher risk than others for malpractice suits, and this is something to be aware of when choosing a subspecialty. In general, surgical specialties are at greater risk of malpractice lawsuits due to the inherently high stakes of surgical operations and the greater potential impact of error. According to a Medscape survey of 4000 physicians in 2017[4], the following medical specialties had the highest self-reported rates of medical malpractice suits, in descending order:

General Surgery
Obstetrics and Gynecology
Otolaryngology (ENT surgery)
Urology
Orthopedic surgery
Plastic surgery
Radiology
Emergency Medicine
Gastroenterology
Anesthesiology

In each of these specialties, over fifty percent of physicians reported being sued in the past, with the highest rates being eighty-five percent in general surgeons and OB-GYN. As is evident from this list, procedural/surgical specialties and particularly OB-GYN (which deals with childbirth, one of the highest stakes moments in life), are at higher risk for malpractice suits. It would be prudent to be aware of the risk of malpractice if you are interested in any medical specialty, but particularly if you foresee a career as a surgeon or proceduralist.

Now what does a malpractice lawsuit actually mean? Malpractice lawsuits are civil suits, brought by a patient against a physician, which put the physician at risk of financial penalty/liability if found to be at fault. It is important to note, though, that these suits alone cannot revoke a physician's license. To lose their license, a physician must show a pattern of negligence and endangerment to patients, and the decision to revoke a license must be made by the state licensing board. Thus, physicians who make an error or are negligent can be held liable/penalized financially, but will typically only be at risk of losing their license if there is a pattern of behavior or an error so egregious that it necessitates revocation of their license for the protection of the public. Typically, malpractice suits will pose only a financial risk to most physicians who are conscientious and well-intentioned but simply made a mistake as any human being may. Some physicians may practice their entire career free of litigation, but many will have to deal with malpractice at some point in their careers.

It is also important to note that physicians do not handle this challenge alone. It is essentially a given in modern American medicine that physicians will obtain malpractice insurance. This is an insurance policy to assist physicians with costs associated with a malpractice suit, from lawyer fees to medical damages to punitive damages. Though not technically required in all states to practice medicine, many hospitals and large medical groups will require physicians to have their own policy or a group policy provided by the organization. Thus, malpractice insurance is essentially ubiquitous for physicians in the US. Though this does not cover all potential costs of a lawsuit, nor does it protect the physician from stress associated with litigation and more severe ramifications like suspension or loss of license, it is a safety net that provides at least some financial protection should a lawsuit arise.

As with any pitfall of life as a physician, don't let this be the main driver of your decision. Weigh this in conjunction with the other elements the career has to offer. Though the risk of malpractice litigation is something all practicing physicians are exposed to, it typically does not detract significantly from the rewards and benefits of the career. In my experience, most physicians practice freely for the benefit of their patients and do not live in fear of legal recourse. Only you can ultimately decide if this risk is a consideration for your future; but most of us accept the reality of malpractice lawsuits and do not consider it a significant deterrent to a fulfilling career in medicine.

Psychological Impacts

The potential psychological impacts of a career as a physician are considerable. Though it can provide significant fulfillment and incredible experiences, the career also carries the potential for overwork, emotional burnout, and depression. Once again, we see the duality of medicine, a pervasive theme in the physician experience. These psychosocial impacts of medicine are significant enough that they warrant dedication of a separate chapter to the discussion of this topic. In the pages that follow, we will assess the psychological and emotional implications (both good and bad) of a career as a physician.

Chapter 14: Psychological and Emotional Impacts of a Career as a Physician

In his classic compilation of fables entitled *The Prophet*, Khalil Gibran said "the deeper that sorrow carves into your being, the more joy you can contain." This beautiful line perfectly summarizes a timeless concept: without the lows of life, the highs would not be nearly as sweet. Few pursuits better capture this vast emotional experience of humanity than the practice of medicine. It comes with some tremendous highs and considerable lows, but a career in medicine undoubtedly creates a broad experience that cannot be replicated elsewhere.

I believe that many of us who pursue a career as a physician seek this very thing—a deep emotional experience attained by caring for other human beings in times of need. This is the very fruit we pursue through years of practice and training, as we know that it bears personal fulfillment and professional gratification. Yet in some ways this is a forbidden fruit, which carries a sinister potential as well. The same opportunities in medical practice which can make us feel such poignant highs can produce bitter lows. When repeated, the cumulative weight of these difficult experiences—of death, loss, morbidity, and mortality—can take a toll on the psyche of the physician. There is potential for considerable psychological repercussions, and these are not to be taken lightly.

This chapter is particularly important, as it touches on topics which are not easily discussed and therefore may be avoided in other forums. Let's explore the significant *positive and negative* psychological impacts of this career to better understand the full experience of the medical trainee and practicing physician.

The Positives

Saving Lives and Relieving Suffering

Perhaps the most common reason to pursue a career as a physician is the desire to save lives. On its surface this notion is too superficial to encapsulate the nuanced experience of a practicing physician; however, it does hold some truth in that sometimes (quite amazingly) we *actually do* save lives.

Take for example the code blue situation that we discussed earlier in Chapter 3, in which a patient is resuscitated and revived after their heart has stopped beating. This is truly an amazing feat of modern medicine, which is nothing short of miraculous when executed successfully. It is not always this dramatic or immediate, but it is true that physicians do save lives. Sometimes it is a primary care physician who identifies a cancerous lung nodule on a screening CT scan in a smoking patient, allowing that nodule to be removed before it grows into a full-blown cancer. Sometimes it is a neurosurgeon evacuating a large brain bleed which would have been fatal if not removed. Sometimes it is a hospitalist treating a patient with a severe infection/sepsis which otherwise would have claimed the patient's life. Sometimes it is a psychiatrist providing the medical care and counseling needed to help a suicidal patient conquer their depression. In these ways and so many others, physicians do save lives. It does not happen for each of us on a daily basis, but it certainly does happen over the course of a career. When it does, the positive feeling is undeniable. This opportunity is an amazing privilege afforded by this unique profession.

It is important to note that just as in the example of the code blue, there are several other team members contributing to the ultimate outcome, helping physicians to save patients in times of need. Nurses, pharmacists, therapists, and many more are in part responsible for a physician's successes. We really do work as a team, and none of our triumphs are achieved alone. This team concept is another particularly rewarding component of a medical career.

Helping Others in Times of Need

Another impactful component of the practice of medicine is helping others in times of need. As medical providers, we are trusted with information and responsibilities which our patients may not even bestow upon their closest loved ones. That bond is sacred, and the provider has the utmost duty to help the patient to the best of their ability. This creates an environment in which the physician can connect with the patient on a deep level, perhaps not easily attainable in other professional fields. Being there for someone in their time of need, helping them fight through and emerge stronger is a powerful experience. Though not every patient interaction will have such an impact, the opportunity to help patients in this way is certainly a positive emotional aspect of this career.

I can think of many instances when I have received unexpected thanks from a patient for the work I have done to help them improve their health and well-being during tough times. We do this daily and dutifully, without a second's hesitation, because this is what we set out to do with our life's work. Often the gratitude for what we do is there but not specifically stated. In those cases, there is still a significant fulfillment that comes with helping a patient and seeing their situation improve. In some cases, though, patients and their loved ones take the time to explicitly thank you, to recognize you for the impact you have made on the patient's life during a particularly challenging time. It usually catches me off guard, if I am being honest, because praise and thanks are not always a common experience and certainly not an expectation. We do our jobs to the best of our ability for the sake of the patient, irrespective of any recognition. But when thanks and heartfelt feelings do come, the emotional effect is awesome. It boosts my spirit and reminds me that despite all the tough times, medical practice is worth it. We are doing good deeds each day and in the process bettering the lives of many of our patients. I typically thank my patients and their families right back, saying "I appreciate you! We don't often get such positive feedback, so it means a lot. Thank you so much for taking the time." Moments like this when we can tangibly feel the impact of our work are a priceless prize in the practice of medicine.

Effecting Positive Change in the Lives of Others

One of the best components of a career as a physician is developing longitudinal, sometimes even lifelong relationships with patients. Particularly in fields with outpatient practice in which chronic diseases are managed, the physician and the patient work together over many years to maintain health and well-being for the patient. In doing so, the physician can help the patient better themselves, imparting knowledge and treatment plans which can effect positive change. Though not easy to achieve by any means, this sort of impact can be very rewarding.

Take, for example, the primary care physician who meets a new patient who is overweight with elevated blood sugar and poorly controlled diabetes. Through long-term medication management, lifestyle changes such as improved diet and exercise, and monitoring for diabetes-related complications, the physician and patient together can change the course of the patient's life. They can achieve weight loss and good blood sugar control, allowing the patient to live a long, healthy, active life. Without such dedicated, diligent intervention from both patient and physician, the patient could live a much more difficult life. It could be fraught with debilitating complications of diabetes such as kidney disease, heart attacks and strokes, or loss of eyesight. Preventing patient suffering, achieving this positive change and thereby increasing patient quality of life, can be something truly special.

Constant Learning and Personal/Professional Growth

A career in healthcare provides the opportunity to constantly learn and grow within the ever-changing world of medical knowledge. One never truly masters all medical science has to offer, as the body of knowledge is simply too vast and is, in fact, always growing. Furthermore, no two patients are the same; though they may present with similar diseases, each patient is unique in their medical pathology as well as their personal and social background. Thus, medicine will provide a constant intellectual challenge throughout one's career. The dynamic nature of the field and its everyday practice is one of the most exciting components of the career. It creates an occupation in which no two days are the same, which helps maintain stimulation and excitement over the years. I firmly believe that among the most rewarding components of any profession are the challenges it provides and the personal growth and fulfillment that come with surpassing these hurdles. Medicine offers an environment which will continually evolve over time, allowing the physician to grow in knowledge and skill, care and compassion, intellectual and emotional capacity.

Opportunity for Innovation

The dynamic landscape of medicine is in large part generated by creative individuals with unique visions, pushing the bounds of medical science. Opportunity for innovation goes hand in hand with a career as a physician and can be one of its most rewarding components for those who wish to pursue it. There are many frontiers for innovation in the medical field, including basic science research, clinical research, epidemiology, medical technology, informatics, public policy, global health, and more. The opportunity for intellectual creativity is inherent to the practice of medicine. By spending years developing specialized knowledge, physicians have a unique vantage point to identify questions that need to be answered and problems that need to be solved. A desire to innovate will not be inherently present for all physicians. Some will focus on clinical practice and being the best physician they can possibly be, which is an honorable and respectable pursuit. But for those who have the interest, for example the MD-PhD running a research lab or the physician with creative ideas they wish to pursue, innovation can become a key component of a medical career. With some inspiration and effort, physicians can pursue medical innovation and thereby find significant professional satisfaction.

The Negatives

While the benefits of a career in medicine are numerous, there are certainly some emotional and psychological downsides to the career which we would be remiss to ignore. Duality once again rears its (sometimes ugly) head. Let's begin with the most obvious: death.

Death/Loss

Each and every profession carries its own pitfalls, as no walk of life is without bumps along the road. But in medicine there is a unique challenge that cannot be avoided, one as sure as the breath that sustains our life itself: death. This is an absolute of any living being's existence and it is surely an absolute of the physician experience. As a shepherd of humanity through the maladies of life, a physician cannot avoid the simple truth that their patients will one day die.

Of course, this absolute truth takes many different forms. Some patients die peacefully in the comfort of their own homes and the company of their loved ones. Others approach death slowly and expectantly, greeting it like an old friend as they pass from this life. But other times death is unexpected and senseless. Sometimes it is shocking and perplexing. Sometimes it is so abrupt that it seems to make no sense at all.

These times are terribly difficult for patients and families, so much so that words cannot do them justice. They bring sorrow, intermingled with anger and regret. The pain I have seen families endure in these moments is enough to break anyone's heart, including those who are there to bear witness (you may recall the story from Chapter 3). There is no doubt in my mind that these moments deeply affect physicians, nurses, and medical professionals alike, no matter how seasoned or "hardened" they may be. Medicine undoubtedly poses many challenges, but perhaps most difficult are these moments when we interface so closely with death. I have felt most helpless in those instances when the tools and skills possessed are not equipped to combat the disease on the other side of the battlefield. Sometimes medicine loses this battle. Sometimes it does not stand a chance. Those times, I must say, are the hardest.

I recall one instance when I felt my medical skillset had nothing to combat the disease we were up against.

I calmly walked down to the ER one afternoon, relatively early in my career as a new attending. I met a pleasant elderly woman, vibrant and sharp, but coming in with a new bout of abdominal pain. She was an immigrant, highly intelligent and vivacious. It was uncanny but her energy reminded me of my own grandmother, who was not terribly different in age. Upon further review of her lab work and vital signs, the patient was sicker than it seemed on the surface. She was presenting to the hospital with signs of sepsis, an inflammatory reaction created by the body in response to an infection, which can be serious and even life-threatening if severe. But in this patient's case, despite her abdominal pain, her labs and imaging did not show any evidence of infection. The underlying cause of her presentation was not clear.

Nevertheless, she was admitted to the hospital for IV fluids, IV antibiotics, and close monitoring, the standard therapy for a patient with sepsis. But within a few hours of arriving at the emergency room, her vital signs began to decline. That night she was transferred to the ICU and started on medicines to maintain her blood pressure. Given her ongoing abdominal pain and a blood test showing a high amount of acid developing in her blood (this is a common phenomenon in critically ill patients), we were concerned for an occult cause of intestinal ischemia, which is essentially inadequate blood flow to the bowels. I consulted a surgeon, as the definitive treatment for severe bowel ischemia is surgery, but her condition was deteriorating quickly. Unfortunately, due to her age and critical status at this point, surgery was deemed a very risky intervention that she likely would not survive. I felt the weight of a potential lost life hovering over me. Though I continued with my work as usual, hustling to get through a busy day caring for many sick patients in addition to her, an ominous feeling lingered within me.

But I had to press on. After lengthy discussions with her family, and in accordance with the wishes she had previously expressed at the time of her admission, we transitioned the patient to comfort-oriented care. This is an approach which aims to minimize pain/suffering and optimize quality of life, with however much time the patient has remaining. The patient's family opted on her behalf to employ this method of care, rather than pursuing heroic measures such as a risky exploratory abdominal surgery in pursuit of an explanation for her critical condition. She was made as comfortable as possible by means of medications and minimizing further interventions, and her immediate family was brought to her bedside. By the next morning, her entire family had arrived, a large group including her husband, children, and grandkids.

When I entered the room and looked around, I felt a strong personal connection to the patient and her family that I did not entirely expect. As physicians we certainly practice empathy but typically do so from a safe distance, as deeper involvement can take an unsustainable emotional toll over time. But this day was different for me—I was choked up and emotional upon entering the room. I steadied myself as I have learned to do over the years, providing a few simple words of support and respect to the patient and family. We had been over the details of her medical course prior, and they understood the situation. This was no longer the time for technical information. It was now time to recognize a wonderful human being whose time on this earth was fading. And just as importantly, it was time to support a loving family through the grief of losing their loved one.

As I stepped out of the room several minutes later, I expected (based on her most recent vital signs and blood work) that she was likely hours away from passing. For one of the first times in my career as a physician, I truly felt the weight of this impending loss almost as if it was my own family. I quickly stepped into the stairwell, only feet away from this room at the back of the ICU, and sat down on the stairs, alone. Tears welled up in my eyes and came rolling down my cheeks. My breath choked in my throat. As someone who has historically had a hard time expressing emotion this way, I was taken aback at my own reaction. Surely, this was a very sad moment for patient, family, and medical providers alike; but it was also a very reasonable and appropriate decision by the family to pursue comfort care for their loved one, sparing her the suffering that can come with a difficult stay in the ICU. And furthermore, this was not nearly my first close encounter with death, as I had been in this situation many times over. So why was I so moved at this moment?

And then it dawned on me, clear as day. I saw my own grandmother in that bed. I saw my own family in that room. The tight-knit group, many of whom had immigrated to this country, who loved their youthful grandmother so dearly—this was very similar to my own experience. And to see such a sudden loss of life—a woman going from independence to passing in a matter of days without a clear explanation—this shook us all to the core.

With years of experience, we learn to deflect the weight of grief in order to preserve ourselves and our ability to practice medicine. But sometimes we feel the true impact of a patient's death as if it were one of our own. Sometimes in those difficult cases which progress quickly without any medical tools to stop the inevitable, we take the burden of the loss on ourselves. Sometimes these losses even feel like personal failures, though almost always they are not. Each time, even when we must move to our next patient seamlessly, the weight of loss is added to the cumulative toll of a physician's emotional experience. This toll, this ledger of loss, is something we all must live with.

I do believe that all physicians are affected by this stress and trauma of death to some degree. It is something we all deal with in our own way. I don't feel that the burden of grief outweighs the positive aspects of a career in medicine, the happy moments with patients and the triumphs we regularly feel. Yet over time, death can leave a lasting impact on the psychological and emotional health of all medical professionals, and physicians are no exception. It is important to be aware of this when considering a medical career.

Patient Morbidity

Along the same lines as loss of life, patient suffering can also take a toll on the provider. A physician's role is to cure disease and relieve symptoms, but at times this cannot be achieved. Sometimes we end up prolonging life, and in doing so we treat patients through their suffering, hoping to mitigate whatever pain or symptoms they have along the way. A fact every medical provider must come to terms with is that patients are sick, plain and simple. We take care of patients with a vast array of diseases. Each of these diseases has the potential to cause patient suffering. We aspire to reduce the burden of disease and thereby mitigate this suffering, and often we do achieve this. This surely brings relief to the patient and fulfillment to the provider. But even in doing so, we witness pain, nausea, shortness of breath, anxiety, and a number of morbidities. These are daily aspects of physician life. We feel for our patients and we strive to help them to the best of our ability. We treat them with clinical care and emotional support, both of which are important remedies. The toll of these encounters is perhaps imperceptible on a daily basis, but it is not to be discounted over the course of a career. It does have an effect over time. Hopefully, the physician can achieve a net positive experience in which helping patients outweighs the burden of suffering traversed along the way. For most physicians I do believe this net positive outcome is the reality; but morbidity is certainly a consideration for the mental and emotional well-being of healthcare providers.

Life Sacrifices

A significant challenge of medical education/training (and sometimes even practice), one which is unavoidable and undeniably difficult, is the amount of life sacrifices that must be made. Much like any other field, mastery of a craft takes time, dedication, and hard work. Though the road to becoming a physician is long, it is probably appropriately long in order to create the skill needed to effectively heal the human body. But in addition to the many years they require, both medical training and practice can put significant demands on a physician's time throughout the process, such that they must sacrifice in other areas of life. As previously discussed, particularly during clinical rotations in med school and residency, medical trainees miss birthdays, weddings, and holidays while working in the hospital. As I like to say, disease doesn't sleep, and the hospital doesn't close. It is a twenty-four/seven institution. This is a simple fact of our lives in medicine: we must ensure our patients are cared for whether it is a Monday morning in April or Christmas morning in December.

This inflexibility in schedule, and the resultant compromise of important life moments, is most pronounced in medical school and residency. If I am honest with myself and you as the reader, this was perhaps the most challenging emotional component of medical training for me. I did not mind working hard for the majority of the year; but missing important life moments took an emotional and psychological toll, as time with family and friends is extremely important to me. These seemingly minor missed moments had a much greater impact on my quality of life than I expected. Certain components of emotional balance and satisfaction are key to longevity in any career. One of those is adequate time to recharge, and for many this is best done through time spent with loved ones. I do feel that every aspiring doctor must eventually acknowledge that attaining their dream takes considerable sacrifice. This is not necessarily inappropriate, as achievement in any realm does require some sacrifice; but one should ensure that this is an acceptable tradeoff to them. This challenge is certainly surmountable, but it is something to be aware of sooner rather than later.

As a career rolls on, the practicing physician does have more autonomy and control over their schedule. Specifically, one can choose specialties that focus on outpatient/clinic-based practice, which allow for freedom on most nights, weekends, and holidays. On the flip side, hospital-based physicians or those who deal with emergencies (such as cardiologists or trauma surgeons) will continue to deal with night and weekend call as well as missed holidays. Overall, the attending lifestyle certainly improves compared to that of a resident in training, but attending physicians do continue to sacrifice life at home to care for their patients. Whether or not this is an issue for you, and to what degree, depends entirely on your personal values. Ultimately, sacrifice is something all physicians (and all professionals for that matter) deal with in some shape or form. It is sufficient to simply be aware that a career as a physician will require sacrifice, as most great things in life do.

Electronic Health Records: The "Pleasures" of Documentation and Billing

We live in a society of quickly growing technology, with advances happening more rapidly than ever before. One of medicine's most consequential technological developments was the widespread adoption of the electronic health record. Though this may seem primitive now, this development occurred within the last few decades and changed the way we practice medicine. Though EHRs have been around longer, legislation such as the Health Information Technology for Economic and Clinical Health (HITECH) Act in 2009[1] have boosted adoption and development of EHRs in the last two decades. With that said, many current physicians trained and practiced in an era when the computer was a non-factor in the delivery of healthcare.

The EHR undoubtedly has significant benefits in information storage and access, reduction of medical error, and communication across medical systems, to name a few. EHRs are integral and beneficial to the medical system. But as is the case with many things in life (and this book), there are two sides of the coin. There have also been some negative outcomes from the technological advancement of EHRs. In particular, the advent of the EHR has created a tremendous burden of documentation and billing for physicians. Data suggest that about half a physician's time is spent on the computer rather than at the bedside delivering direct patient care[2]. This extra time is typically spent reviewing the chart, documenting the encounter, coding diagnoses, and billing in the EHR. Anecdotally, I would tend to agree with this fifty percent number; though it does vary by specialty and individual provider, it is reasonable to estimate that many physicians spend about half their working hours utilizing the medical record.

I can confidently say that most physicians pursued medicine to apply their hard-earned skills to direct patient care in order to benefit the patient. We dreamed of interacting with people, not computers, when we imagined our life's work. Though direct patient care is still a large part of what we do, a huge amount of time is spent on EHRs ensuring that our documentation is up to code and our billing is complete, so that we can receive appropriate reimbursement from insurance companies and health plans. Though a necessary component of our healthcare system (and though I cannot offer an immediate solution), this burden almost always reduces physician satisfaction. Studies show that the amount of time physicians spend with patients has not changed significantly over the last few decades[3] despite the advent of the EHR. Therefore, increased time spent on documentation and billing means longer work hours for physicians, which in turn decreases satisfaction and increases the likelihood of burnout (more details on this topic in Chapter 15). The burden of increased tasks and responsibilities imposed by the EHR is a challenge we must all navigate in the world of modern medicine.

Performance Incentives/Relative Value Units

Along similar lines as electronic burdens, today's physicians are increasingly bound by a need to demonstrate the quantity and quality of their performance. Relative value units (RVUs) are measures of physician productivity, and directly affect compensation in many payment models. RVUs are a means of measuring and comparing different services rendered by physicians, as not all services are equal. They consider multiple factors including the time, expertise, and resources required to provide the service. Thus, RVUs create a system which can measure the relative "value" (as it pertains to compensation) of different medical services, such as a surgery versus a primary care visit. Subsequently, a conversion factor (dollars per RVU) is applied to determine compensation.

Though essential to the finances of many healthcare systems, RVUs can create an extrinsic system of motivation, in which motivation is derived from an external factor such as a financial reward. Logic would indicate that physicians may end up focusing at least in part on demonstrating productivity rather than simply providing excellent patient care. Though there is a lot of sense and utility to the system of compensation based on RVUs, it does create the possibility of poor incentives (quantity rather than quality), which ultimately may affect care and lead to less professional satisfaction for the physician.

Meanwhile, quality performance measures also make good sense in many ways, as they hold physicians accountable for patient outcomes rather than incentivizing them to see more patients. But they can also have some detrimental effects in terms of increased burden of documentation and making physicians feel that they are beholden to metrics rather than patients. Inevitably, physicians do feel burdened by additional oversight and reduced autonomy. It is not that physicians do not want to strive for high quality; most do, as they are motivated intrinsically by a desire to do their best and to do right by their patients. But a need to *demonstrate* quality of performance through documentation, billing, and metrics can detract from the joy of applying medical knowledge for the betterment of the patient (the reason most of us pursued medicine in the first place). It is a fine line that the healthcare system walks currently, between physician wellness and incentivizing patient outcomes/metrics for cost-effectiveness and quality of care. But this is something physicians will need to adjust to, as "value-based care" (care which derives payment from patient outcomes rather than number of patients seen) is becoming more common.

The burden of the EHR—documentation, billing, metrics, and RVUs—can create a system in which the physician is acting with less autonomy and less ability to focus on what matters most: connecting with patients and providing outstanding care. It is no secret that these factors contribute to physician burnout and negative emotional outcomes. We will discuss the topic of burnout further in the pages to come. In the meantime, be aware that the modern physician will need to navigate the electronic challenges of a medical career, while the healthcare system at large will need to determine how to best use technology for the betterment of patients *and* physicians. It is certainly a work in progress, but I am optimistic about the future.

Burnout

Though there are several positive components of a career in medicine which can promote happiness and fulfillment, there exist more sinister components of the profession which can lead to frustration, dissatisfaction, and even depression. The term *burnout* has been coined to describe this phenomenon. It is not necessarily specific to medicine, but it bears particular relevance to the field. Burnout has become increasingly common in medical professionals and it is something which shouldn't be taken lightly. There is no easy solution to burnout, but a significant amount of work is ongoing to both understand it and develop strategies to mitigate it. It is a common topic of discussion in the medical world today because of its significant prevalence and impact.

Burnout is such an important issue that I found it best to dedicate an entire chapter to it. I am by no means an expert, but I will provide an overview of burnout, the factors that drive it, and some strategies to combat it. An understanding of the issue at hand and the factors which contribute to it will make you more prepared to face it in the future. Hopefully this knowledge will help you to prevent, identify, and mitigate burnout in any walk of life.

Chapter 15: Burnout

Burnout is a term that was initially used in health care in the 1970's to describe the phenomenon of work-related stress causing negative psychological and emotional effects on the healthcare professional[1]. The term has evolved over time, taking on powerful colloquial and academic meanings. It is becoming nearly ubiquitous in conversations regarding the healthcare profession. As we come to better understand and describe it, burnout has become a topic of immense discussion in the medical field.

What is Burnout?

Burnout is a specific form of occupational stress leading to physical and emotional exhaustion and loss of fulfillment from work. It is precipitated by work-related systems, environments, and stressors. Its cardinal features are loss of energy/feelings of exhaustion, mental detachment/negative feelings towards one's works, and decreased professional effectiveness[2]. Burnout has been shown to negatively affect physician performance, increasing error and decreasing patient satisfaction[3]. Perhaps even more importantly, it can be accompanied by anxiety, depression, and even suicidality. Though it is not this severe for all those affected, burnout in any form can take a considerable toll on any individual who experiences it.

Burnout is indicative of a disturbance in emotional and mental health for the individual it affects. On a broader scale though, it is symptomatic of disease at the systemic level, representing the failings of our healthcare system to maintain physician well-being. The inherent nature of medicine unfortunately does create a high risk for burnout: the physical and mental tax of long hours and grueling work; interfacing with suffering and loss of life; and a system which has historically favored physicians "toughing it out" rather than prioritizing their mental and physical well-being. Based on these factors it is not surprising that physician burnout is a significant issue within the medical field.

With that said, a large amount of scholarly work is being done on burnout to better understand its root causes and its solutions. Burnout is an entity which we are coming to better understand as awareness of the scale and the impact of the problem is growing steadily. Hopefully this work will help our field combat this destructive phenomenon. But it is incumbent upon current and future physicians to remain aware of the issue and vigilant of its signs and symptoms. Awareness may help us combat burnout, for ourselves and our peers alike.

How Prevalent is Burnout?

The main challenge with describing the prevalence of the problem is the difficulty in specifically defining burnout. Particularly for research purposes, burnout is a tricky thing to define as it is multifactorial and can present in many ways. As discussed, there is an overarching condition of burnout which manifests as a lack of satisfaction with work due to its inherent conditions. Burnout also can be defined as having subcomponents such as emotional exhaustion, depersonalization with work, and low personal achievement or effectiveness[4]. Finally, it can have accompanying symptoms such as anxiety and depression. Burnout is a complex and multifaceted entity and therefore it can be difficult to define and study.

Nevertheless, there have been several studies assessing the prevalence of burnout among physicians. A recent systematic review evaluated 182 studies assessing burnout and different combinations of the above sub-definitions[4]. The review reported that overall burnout prevalence in the studies evaluated "ranged from 0% to 80.5%. Meanwhile, emotional exhaustion, depersonalization, and low personal accomplishment prevalence ranged from 0% to 86.2%, 0% to 89.9%, and 0% to 87.1%, respectively." Quite notably, these are huge statistical ranges and are therefore difficult to interpret. The review found significant heterogeneity in burnout definitions and symptom scoring tools used to define burnout, making it nearly impossible to accurately calculate a composite burnout prevalence. What is clear though is that a significant portion of these studies reported considerable burnout prevalence, with some topping fifty percent as noted above.

Due to the inherent difficulty of defining burnout in a rigorous manner (an issue which will likely improve in coming years with a growing body of research), simple surveys may be a more feasible means of assessing burnout in the medical community. Such data also do exist; though less objective than defining burnout based on symptom scores/tools in a rigorous research study, these data are still meaningful because they describe both physician perception and experience.

A survey conducted in 2018 by the AMA received responses from over 15,000 physicians in twenty-nine medical specialties[5]. Overall, forty-two percent of physicians were found to have burnout, which was down from fifty-one percent the year prior. The medical specialties with the highest prevalence of burnout were as follows:

Critical care: 48%
Neurology: 48%
Family medicine: 47%
Obstetrics and gynecology: 46%
Internal medicine: 46%
Emergency medicine: 45%

Meanwhile, the specialties with the lowest burden of burnout were the following:

Plastic surgery: 23%
Dermatology: 32%
Pathology: 32%
Ophthalmology: 33%
Orthopedics: 34%

As is evident from these self-reported physician data, burnout is highly prevalent regardless of specialty. Even the specialties with the lowest prevalence may have about a quarter of their physicians affected, which is not an insignificant number. There is a considerable burden of this phenomenon within the physician community, which is undoubtedly consequential to physician well-being. It therefore behooves the medical field to better understand this issue, increase awareness, and combat it as best we can.

Only by raising awareness of burnout can we advance our understanding of it and direct efforts toward effecting change.

Future generations of aspiring physicians deserve to understand such challenges which face their future profession as a whole and may also stand as personal hurdles along their path. Be aware, be informed, be powerful. With this knowledge you will be better equipped to make decisions about your future career, while having the vigilance to identify and combat burnout should it ever be an issue you face along your own journey.

What Causes Burnout?

Perhaps the most important step in combatting burnout is understanding what drives it. There are many answers to the question of what causes burnout, as the experience is personal and heterogenous with different causative factors in each individual. Still, there are some repeated themes and issues which are common drivers of physician burnout.

According to the same survey conducted by the AMA in 2018, an unreasonable burden of "bureaucratic tasks" was the top reported cause of physician burnout[5]. Over the years, the art and practice of medicine have trended away from critical thinking and direct patient contact to more regulated, less autonomous processes. This trend can make physicians feel like a cog in a wheel. While most recognize the benefit of increased consistency of medical practice and diligent documentation in the EHR, there is no denying that these changes place an additional mental burden on physicians (recall Chapter 14). Many physicians, including myself, imagined their career in medicine filled with patient-centered encounters, opportunities to think critically and apply skills while helping *people*. When that vision morphs into a reality of hours spent in front of *computers* documenting, billing, and checking bureaucratic boxes, the joy can drain from an already challenging profession.

Physicians in the 2018 AMA survey also reported the following as top causes of burnout: spending too many hours at work, lack of respect, increased computerization of practice, and insufficient compensation[5]. Other reports have identified loss of autonomy as an additional driver of physician burnout. Many of these factors go hand in hand with increased bureaucratic tasks. Physicians no longer practice at the height of their skills when they are burdened by electronic tasks and expectations designed by organizations. Furthermore, a generational transition to the use of EHRs has disillusioned an earlier cohort of physicians who came from an era focused on direct patient contact. The demands of documentation and billing tether physicians to computers and not to patients, while increasing organizational scrutiny and individual workload.

Finally, a significant driver of physician burnout can simply be the emotional demand which comes with being a healthcare provider. Carrying the burden of death and disease is hard no matter how solid the foundational support systems are. Some physicians may encounter hopelessness associated with being unable to reverse some of the underlying issues which drive suffering and disease: poverty, socioeconomic disparities, and lack of access to necessary treatment including preventative healthcare. When viewed in this light, the battle of medicine can seem like a steep hill to traverse, leaving some providers emotionally exhausted.

How Do We Combat Burnout?

As burnout is such a heterogeneous entity, with varying manifestations in unique individuals, it is also a complex problem to treat and prevent. A basic approach which has been proposed and is starting to be employed in medical systems as well as residency programs is the use of mindfulness practices and other stress-reduction techniques such as yoga or meditation. These are worthwhile endeavors with some utility for those who wish to employ them. Mindfulness is an evidence-based technique to mitigate work-related stress, although more robust research is required[6-8]. With that said, these approaches alone are insufficient as they are symptomatic treatments which do not address the underlying causes of burnout. They are more useful as an adjunct to what is truly needed: more profound systemic change.

To address the root causes of burnout, one significant change which may provide benefit is structural alterations to EHRs to make them more adapted to physician workflow and efficiency. It is in the best interest of our profession to create electronic systems which augment physicians' ability to process information and administer effective care, rather than burdening them with additional responsibilities and encumbering physician-patient interaction. Furthermore, systemic and perhaps even regulatory changes to the demands of documentation could improve physician workflow, reduce work hours, and thereby mitigate burnout. Additional considerations which could improve physician workflow in the future would be enhanced interoperability of EHRs[5] (which would allow providers to view records from other systems with much less effort) as well as artificial intelligence capabilities (which could potentially assist with documentation and identification of key patient information in the health record).

We know electronic burdens have the potential to increase burnout and are thus a possible area of improvement. But what other changes can be made to help physicians prevent and reduce burnout? Physicians reported in 2018 that reduced work hours and opportunities for education/personal growth are factors that would reduce burnout[5]. Reducing work hours would undoubtedly be a considerable challenge; but as discussed above, altering the role/function of EHRs to help rather than hinder physician workflow is a potential improvement which could save time. Furthermore, systems putting less emphasis on productivity (which thereby increases physician workload) could help maintain physician work hours at a reasonable level. Meanwhile, opportunities for personal growth come in the form of educational conferences, courses, and involvement in professional societies. Helping physicians pursue such experiences depends upon making those pursuits not only allowed but encouraged within the work environment. It is incumbent upon employers and health systems to provide physicians with time and financial resources that support continuing education and opportunities for professional growth. This will help promote the intellectual engagement that made medicine such an exciting field in the first place. With healthcare organizations becoming increasingly aware of burnout in this era of modern medicine, they will need to focus on these interventions and more to help mitigate this issue in the future.

Finally, an important intervention in preventing physician burnout and its symptomatic outcomes, including depression and anxiety, is the encouragement and availability of mental health services for medical professionals. There is a historic stigma associated with the use of mental health services which exists across all fields. But please let me take this moment to say that this stigma is completely unfounded. It should be combatted with a vengeance, as it discourages individuals in need to seek the healthcare that they deserve. Mental health should be viewed no differently than physical health in terms of its importance to the effective functioning of the human body. Just as we would never discourage an individual with heart or lung disease from seeking medical treatment, individuals suffering from depression, anxiety, or other mental health ailments should never be discouraged from seeking the medical help they need.

The irony is that the stigma with mental health and the associated hesitance to seek professional guidance exists among medical professionals just as much as it does in the general public. This trend is improving as awareness of mental health issues within healthcare and the necessity of treatment is on the rise; nevertheless, physicians are not always willing or ready to seek help. Though they are as well-versed in the importance of appropriate mental health treatment as a mechanic is with an oil-change, some physicians are not immune from the stigma and the resultant reluctance to seek that very same treatment. One can understand the hesitation of a highly functioning professional to admit that they need help in this very vulnerable and personal manner. The reluctance is likely worsened by concerns over employers or state licensing boards restricting a physician's ability to practice. In most cases though, seeking mental health treatment will not be a threat to a physician's license unless the issue impairs their ability to practice medicine safely. In this more extreme case, it is to the benefit of doctor and patient that the physician seeks out help and treatment prior to continuing to practice. Most of the time this will not be the case, and the medical provider will be allowed to seek support without jeopardizing their career. Ultimately, this stigma and reluctance must be slowly overturned, as they come at a detriment to the mental health of the medical community.

Among physicians surveyed in 2018, only about thirty to forty percent of physicians experiencing burnout (varying by medical specialty) sought professional help to address it[5]. Physicians are by and large highly functioning individuals who had to employ resilience and perseverance in the face of difficult conditions during their medical education and training to succeed. But perhaps these same skills are risk factors for ignoring mental health symptoms, for avoidance of seeking help and rather trying to "stick it out."

Healthcare employers must make treatment and counseling through psychologists/psychiatrists available and readily accessible to medical professionals. By providing robust systems with easy pathways to find help, while encouraging struggling providers to seek support when needed, healthcare systems can truly make a difference. Such changes will allow the negative mental health outcomes of burnout to be identified and combated as early and effectively as possible.

Burnout is a prevalent and important issue but, ultimately, it does not define the pervasive experience of the practicing physician. Aspiring medical professionals reading this text or encountering other information on burnout should not be discouraged from pursuing their dreams within the medical field. As we have discussed throughout this book so far, a career as a physician is excellent in many ways: intellectual stimulation, interpersonal interaction, personal and professional satisfaction, the ability to touch the lives of others in a uniquely impactful way. The inherent value of a career in medicine will never be completely outweighed by the challenges.

Yet, I encourage readers to be aware of the issues, such as provider burnout, which face our field today. Arm yourself with knowledge. Throughout this book, you have trained yourself for a future in medicine by encountering and interpreting vital information. In reading it you are strengthening your knowledge of the medical field and the experience of practicing within it. Just as a runner's countless hours spent pounding the pavement will help him cross the finish line, time spent turning the pages of this book will ultimately make you stronger and more prepared for your future career.

In the final section of this book, I would like to offer some reflections from my career in the medical field: two key emotional moments in my undergrad experience which encapsulate my premedical journey; and more recently, my experience with perhaps the biggest and most consequential event of the twenty-first century—the COVID-19 pandemic.

Part V: Postscript

Chapter 16: A Reflection on COVID-19 – What We Have Learned from the Global Pandemic

Novel Coronavirus. Sars-COV2. COVID-19. Delta. Mu. Omicron. Many names, one devastating and world-altering disease. Who could have predicted such a catastrophic medical phenomenon would literally change the face of history and the world as we know it?

If a friend had come to you saying that they had a vision of the future, and in that vision a new virus would infect hundreds of millions of people in each corner of the world, killing millions along the way, changing everything from social interaction to global economics—what would have been your response?

No way, that's crazy. That could not happen in this era of modern medicine. Not to mention, since when were you, my friend, a psychic who can see the future?

What if someone else had come to you saying they had the same vision (amazingly), only they had seen further along? They had seen a vaccine developed within nine months of the pandemic's origin, delivered and administered to millions throughout the world, saving countless lives. *No way,* you would say again. *Vaccines and clinical trials take longer to develop than that. Not possible!*

If a third, equally gifted individual had the same premonition and told you that doctors, nurses, and medical professionals across the world had stepped up, risking their lives in service of others, what would be your response? In that case you might say, *Okay. I can believe that. That is the heart and soul of medicine: to rise to the occasion when called upon, to selflessly serve, and to heal fellow citizens. That is what this profession does. That I can believe.*

In the unprecedented year of 2020, one unmatched in modern history, the impossible and unthinkable happened: all the above. As a result of the COVID-19 virus, modern medicine—and our society itself—changed drastically. So, what have we learned from it all and how does it impact your future career as a physician? In the pages that follow, we will reflect on what has occurred and consider what is now to come: the changes in healthcare in the wake of this devastating pandemic.

My Reflection on COVID-19

One sunny morning in early January of 2020, I stroll into our hospitalist workroom at 8:00 AM, the time of our daily morning huddle. I greet my fellow hospitalists, colleagues who I have loved getting to know over the course of my first year as an attending. We all settle in as usual, looking over our patient lists and getting ready to distribute the overnight admissions. Then the silence is broken by a question I will never forget.

"Did everyone hear about this new virus, from Wuhan in China?" one of my colleagues asks, with none of the urgency or gravity which we now associate with the virus. "It's been on the news."

My ears immediately perk up, and I quickly look up from the list of patients I am combing over, internally deliberating on some clinical decisions to be made that day. "No, I haven't actually. What's that all about?"

This is the first time I hear of the highly contagious and quite deadly virus we now know as COVID-19. It is a fresh news story that is just developing, merely an interesting piece of information from a land (but not a galaxy) far, far away. We consider this simply international news, undoubtedly intriguing but with little to no tangible impact on our lives here at home. Our discussion that morning is certainly memorable, but it is perfunctory as so little is known about the virus at that time.

Fast forward to only two months later. I am working on service in the hospital again on a weekday evening in mid-March. The world has been taken by storm over the last month by growing news of the same virus, which is now sweeping across the world as a global pandemic. Still, the tangible effects of this virus are limited for me. I feel great empathy for my medical sisters and brothers fighting this pandemic tooth and nail in New York City, and even greater sadness for the patients already losing their lives on American soil and throughout the world. We are not yet seeing cases in the hospital in San Diego though, and thus the threat remains in some ways conceptual. But we know COVID is coming, and we are bracing for impact. I feel more angst than anything—a desire to contribute, to help my medical peers combat this pandemic sooner rather than later. Yet still we wait. The feeling in the air is eerie and ominous.

I walk into the room of a patient I have just admitted. As I am following up on his clinical condition and symptoms, the TV catches my eye. The US president is addressing the nation, announcing that COVID-19 has been deemed a national emergency. The US will be implementing a travel ban to Europe, during which Americans will no longer be allowed leisure travel across the Atlantic.

Wow, I think. *That is something else. A travel ban? This thing is really taking off.*

I know the impact this disease is having, and I understand the threat it poses, but somehow this simple travel ban drives the point home even further. Perhaps it hits home as I think of my friend who is overseas visiting Europe at that moment, and I wonder if he will make it home safely. The virus is not only affecting lives, but also changing how the international community interacts and behaves. The impacts seem to be taking on a broader scale.

This thing is for real, I think. *COVID is no joke. It's here to stay.*

Within the next few days, I cancel my upcoming international vacation, which had been planned for months and was a huge source of excitement for my wife and me. It is all-hands-on-deck at my hospital and within my physician group. We know the COVID surge is on its way, and we need everyone ready to fight the impending battle. While I must admit I am disappointed about my lost travel plans, I know this is much more important. I am gladly willing to serve.

Meanwhile, societal behaviors change quickly and drastically. A stay-at-home order is issued in California. Most of my friends and family responsibly begin what is now being referred to as "quarantine" but, in reality, is social isolation at home. (Quarantine is isolation imposed on those who were exposed to an infectious disease or traveled from somewhere at risk, whereas isolation is preventative for those without exposure).

For the next several weeks I isolate at home with only my partner, not seeing friends or family but continuing to work in the hospital as usual. We are now admitting and treating COVID-positive patients, and plenty of them. There is much uncertainty in this early stage of the pandemic: limited personal protective equipment (PPE, a medical provider's defense against the virus) which may be depleted at any time; an incomplete understanding of the medical treatment of this new disease; the constant threat of rising and overwhelming patient numbers as is being seen in other cities across the globe; and the unavoidable fear of the unknown. The anxiety is palpable in the hospital, on COVID and non-COVID units alike. Nevertheless, each day I witness the bravery and resolve of medical professionals—physicians, nurses, therapists, pharmacists, case managers, and more—all caring for patients in the hospital without a moment's hesitation. It is impressive to see that despite the highly stressful and challenging circumstances, the medical profession does not flinch in the face of danger. *Bring it on*, we say. *Let's do this.*

The weeks turn into months as the pandemic drones on, without anything to break the monotonous and now rote anxiety of caring for COVID-19 patients at work while isolating at home during time off. One day, I walk down to the emergency room to admit a patient who almost certainly has COVID. At this point, we still do not have N95 masks for our encounters with COVID or suspected-COVID patients (to no fault of our hospital, but rather a systemic and nationwide shortage of this medical necessity). I review the patient's vital signs, labs, and imaging. She has a fever of 102 degrees and a heart rate of 130, glaring signs of an ongoing infection. Her respiratory status is tenuous, as she is currently on a high-flow oxygen delivery device but still having borderline blood oxygen levels. Her blood work is highly consistent with COVID, though her actual COVID test is not yet back, as our current testing methods take hours to days to result. I pull up her x-ray only to see a familiar result: cotton-like spots filling both sides of her lungs, or "bilateral interstitial opacities" as well call them in medicine. These often (but not always) indicate infection; when considered in the context of her other clinical and diagnostic findings, this imaging is almost certainly indicative of pneumonia from COVID-19.

I dawn the appropriate PPE (at that time a surgical mask, gown, gloves, and face shield) and enter the patient's room. She is showing clear signs of respiratory distress, with fast and labored breathing. She is also significantly confused and able to provide only limited answers to my questions. I quickly perform a focused physical exam and assessment of her vitals in the room. As soon as I am done, I remove my PPE and step back into the hallway. Hands thoroughly washed, I immediately write admission orders to the ICU and call my pulmonary critical care colleague. With the high-flow oxygen device, this patient is on nearly maximal respiratory support short of a ventilator; at that time in the pandemic, we were not using non-invasive positive pressure ventilation (commonly known as CPAP or BiPAP) on COVID patients. Given that she is not yet improving with high-flow oxygen, medical experience tells me that she will require intubation and support with a ventilator to survive.

Within minutes, my pulmonary colleague is at the bedside evaluating the patient. He agrees with my assessment and feels that the patient needs to be intubated. Very soon the patient is placed on a ventilator. She is admitted to the ICU and started on supportive therapy for COVID-19. We do not yet have focused antiviral therapies for this disease. The patient undergoes a long hospital course. Given her deterioration and respiratory failure severe enough to require intubation, the pulmonary critical care team takes over for me. I return to care for my other patients, many of whom also have COVID but have staved off the most severe stages of respiratory failure. I am as busy as ever and certainly exhausted, but I keep pushing on knowing my team, my hospital, and my patients need me. Despite the tough times, I take some solace and pride in knowing that my contributions to fighting the pandemic are meaningful. We are helping people and saving lives in the process, and this will forever be something to be thankful for.

Weeks later, I open the same patient's chart to check on her clinical status and progression as I have been doing periodically since her admission. Each time I do this for my sickest patients, I experience a momentary surge of anxiety that our efforts will have failed, and my patient will have passed. This time, unfortunately but not surprisingly, my fears are confirmed: the patient has passed away. Despite all our care and everything medical science currently has to offer in response to this disease, COVID ultimately prevails. I take a moment to send my thoughts and best wishes to the deceased patient and her family. Sadly, she is yet another casualty among thousands (and now millions) during this terrible pandemic.

A few months down the line in fall of 2020, our therapies for COVID-19 have slightly advanced (we are now using steroids and an antiviral medication called remdesivir) and our patients are surviving hospitalization at a higher rate. At the same time, patients are now flowing through our doors in much greater numbers; the virus is taking hold and we are amid a much bigger surge than we initially experienced in the spring. I admit a young man in his mid-thirties, who had the poor fortune of contracting COVID during his recent travels. He is fit and otherwise healthy, so he should have a great chance of recovery from the virus. Initially he is on a minimal amount of oxygen, only two liters at the time of admission to the hospital. But within forty-eight hours, his respiratory status severely declines, and he is escalated to the same high-flow oxygen delivery device that my previous patient required. He is young and healthy, but he is gravely ill from COVID-19.

"Doc, I'm going to survive this right?" he asks me on the third day of his hospitalization. My belief is that he will, so I answer accordingly. But I must also be realistic and honest, as is my duty to the patient. I inform him that there is a decent chance that he further worsens and needs additional respiratory support with a ventilator. I do think he will pull through, but I can't be certain. He is critically ill and there is no escaping that truth. All I can tell him with certainty is that we will do everything in our power to treat and support him through this. Other than that, we can only hope for the best.

COVID is unpredictable in the lives that it claims. One of the most difficult things is knowing we can only offer the maximal medical therapy available, and the rest is up to the virus and the patient's immune system. We cannot cure this disease in every patient. My patient understands and appreciates my honesty, but he is visibly shaken by the response. I suspect this is the first time he has ever had to face his own mortality. These are unprecedented times creating previously unthinkable situations.

"I can only imagine how hard this is," I tell him. "But I will do everything I can to get you through this. We must remain positive." It is tough to see someone so young and otherwise healthy now so sick from this disease. I picture myself or one of my friends in his shoes. It is a difficult thought to bear. I push it away from my mind, refocusing my attention and effort on supporting him medically and emotionally—on helping him survive.

Weeks later, after a lengthy and tumultuous hospital course, the patient has finally recovered. To my huge relief, his vitals have improved, and he has been weaned off of oxygen. Based on where he was during his peak level of illness, he is one of the lucky ones. His course could easily have gone the other way. He is fortunate to be alive. The patient leaves the hospital and rejoins his family at home, but he is very weak and still short of breath. It will likely take him weeks to months to recover, and his lung capacity may never be the same again. Still, we give thanks that we were able to see this one through and that this young man was able to return home, alive.

At the time I initially wrote this reflection in early 2021, we were still absolutely in the thick of the pandemic. As a matter of fact, the number of COVID patients in my hospital had never been higher. We had nearly one hundred COVID cases in our hospital and over four hundred in our entire hospital system. We were in the middle of California's second stay at home order. Times were tough but the vaccine was close on the horizon, providing more hope than we previously had at any point during this trying ordeal. The winter progressed and our numbers eventually doubled: we reached two hundred COVID patients in my hospital alone. Through it all we kept slogging, kept working as hard as we could to prevent as much death as possible—and hopefully to survive it all ourselves.

Now we have seen two more waves brought on by fierce and ruthless variants whose names are seared in our minds and the pages of medical history: delta and omicron. It seems the pandemic has taken on its own life and personality, evolving with time and posing new challenges every few months. We continue to deal with this disease that only a few years ago did not exist, at least for our species in this form. But our vaccines continue to do tremendous good, and our therapies continue to evolve and improve. I am hopeful.

The end feels near, but no one can be certain when we will be through this all. All we know for certain is that we are not done yet. There is more work to do, more lives to be saved (and sadly lost) before this is all said and done. It has been the experience of a lifetime, but not the type you hope for and certainly not one you ever wish to repeat. In the simplest terms it has been something of a collective nightmare for humanity. My hope is that sometime soon, we will all wake up.

Changes in Healthcare Due to COVID-19

The face of humanity and healthcare have changed dramatically as a result of the COVID-19 virus. Next, let's consider the how the pandemic has altered the American medical system and the experience of the practicing physician.

Balancing Personal Health Risk against the Opportunity to Serve Humanity

One thing that has become easily apparent throughout the COVID-19 pandemic is that physicians and other healthcare workers alike are at risk of exposure to infectious diseases throughout their professional careers. As discussed previously in Chapter 13, the greatest health risk of this profession lies in exposure to infectious diseases. The risk of such diseases could be no more apparent than it is during a global pandemic. COVID-19 is the pandemic to rule them all.

Physicians, nurses, and other healthcare workers have sadly lost their lives to COVID. Yet across the globe, medical professionals continue to put themselves in harm's way to protect and treat others in times of need. Two things have been clear to me during this process. First, the health risk during a career as a physician is non-trivial; it is overall fairly low, but it is greater than I had previously realized. There is a very real possibility that we will deal with other public health/infectious disease crises throughout our careers, during which we will have to assume the risk required to treat our patients. There is no escaping this risk, however minor or significant it may be. Second, I have realized that this risk is not a deterrent for me personally, nor does it seem to be one for my colleagues in this profession. We all continue doing our jobs to the best of our abilities, and in some ways derive even more fulfillment from stepping up during times of crisis. For me, though the pandemic has undoubtedly been scary, the experience has felt like an opportunity to rise to the occasion, to put my training to use in service of others. Though it has been a terrible burden on society, I have tried to find a silver lining by viewing the pandemic as a chance to give back to the world in a deeply impactful way. This has allowed me to stay positive and push forward through these tough times.

The bravery, selflessness, and desire to serve others that define the medical profession have never been more apparent than during the COVID-19 pandemic. I have seen these virtues in countless medical professionals alongside me in the trenches and worldwide in the stories I have read and heard. This indomitable spirit will continue to pervade medicine, making it one of life's most exciting and fulfilling professional pursuits.

Innovation: From Testing to Vaccines

Another feature of the COVID-19 pandemic which has been nothing short of remarkable has been the level of collaboration and innovation which have occurred throughout the medical community. It is amazing to realize that so recently this virus was unbeknownst to mankind, yet within a few months we developed assays for accurate testing. New therapies were studied and implemented only months later. And most amazing of all, less than a year into the pandemic we saw the development and use of multiple vaccines with remarkably high efficacy and very solid safety profiles.

The world of science banded together like never before in the pursuit of a defense against this global catastrophe. This flurry of scientific activity has to excite you—how could it not? It represents the incredibly dynamic nature of medicine. Diseases are always evolving, as is our understanding of them and the human body. Coupled with the active minds and energetic bodies of the scientific community, this ever-changing environment creates an exhilarating field in which to work. For anyone who aspires to be a lifelong learner, or to themselves push the limits of knowledge and innovation, medicine is an outstanding opportunity to meet these goals. As dreadful as this pandemic has been, claiming an unfathomable number of lives, it has revealed the great assets mankind possesses: curiosity of mind, tremendous problem-solving skills, and the ability to adapt and collaborate for the common good. The silver lining of innovation has poised us to hopefully conquer the beast that is COVID-19 soon, on the backs of our brave medical professionals armed with evolving treatments and timely vaccines.

Telemedicine

Another one of the most dynamic facets of humankind is our communication and the ability of technology to augment it. The field of medicine has been tracking the technological progression of the communications industry, albeit more slowly than a tech-giant such as Apple or Google. But with widespread adoption of EHRs over the last two decades and increasing ability to communicate digitally, telemedicine has been growing as an important entity in our field. Then the COVID pandemic hit, and that growth was put into overdrive.

Telemedicine is exactly what it sounds like based on its root words "tele" and "medicine." It is medical care provided by a physician or other provider remotely instead of in-person, via either telephone or video call. It has been employed previously in fields from primary care to even critical care, with intensivists covering hospitals in rural areas via video calling. Since the beginning of the COVID pandemic though, the application of telemedicine has increased exponentially. With the need for social distancing and reduced in-person encounters, a significant portion of outpatient medical care was transitioned to telemedicine during the early pandemic. In my medical group for example, a large amount of outpatient care in clinics was provided via telephone and video visits; meanwhile, more urgent medical issues requiring in-person evaluation were addressed either in clinics, urgent cares, or emergency rooms depending on the clinical scenario. Even within the hospital, to reduce frequency of contact with stable, COVID-positive patients, some encounters by physicians and other medical professionals were transitioned to video visit, via iPad for example. Though this practice has not persisted in my institution for inpatient care, it did demonstrate that telemedicine can be effectively utilized even for hospitalized patients if needed. In swift and efficient fashion, medical systems had to adapt and innovate to use telemedicine as a tool for providing care while maintaining both patient and provider safety as much as possible. In the outpatient setting, telemedicine continues to be a significant part of the workflow for many medical groups. Put simply, telemedicine is here to stay.

After the significant uptick in the use of technology to provide medical care due to the pandemic, there is sure to be continued adoption of telemedicine going forward. In the business sector, many companies have adapted, realizing there is utility and perhaps even benefit to employees working from home. Similarly, medical groups will continue to adapt, utilizing telemedicine when safe and effective. For a rising generation of young physicians who are skilled in the use of technology, this will be a relatively easy transition. There will certainly be some pain points with this process: maintaining the personal patient-physician connection remotely, determining the limitations of telemedicine and the situations in which traditional medical visits are needed, and optimizing communication with the patient, to name a few. But ultimately, telemedicine will be a tool which helps advance the field of medicine. It may be of benefit to patients who prefer to conduct some of their medical care remotely, rather than in the confines of a clinic (and waiting room). Each successive generation is increasingly on-the-go, resulting in increasing utility for remote communication. Telemedicine is no longer the future of healthcare; it has become the present, and its growth has been significantly accelerated by COVID-19.

Concluding Thoughts on COVID-19

Medicine and the world as we know it have been permanently changed by the COVID pandemic. There is no way around that. The experience will be indelible in our minds and the effects will be pervasive and long-lasting. From the healthcare changes already discussed above, to caring for patients with this new disease and its potential long-term effects, to mental health issues which may arise due to social isolation or trauma suffered as a result of the pandemic, the challenges that result from COVID-19 will be numerous. We will not soon forget this life-changing experience; but through resilience and a zest for tackling the next challenge that arises, we will emerge from this experience stronger and more closely bonded than ever. The medical profession is incredible in that it provides the opportunity to directly contribute to society by battling its public health challenges on the front lines. In your career as a physician, should you choose to pursue one, similar challenges will undoubtedly surface. And just like those who came before, you will rise to the occasion and face them head on.

This spirit of bravely facing any challenge perfectly captures the heart of the medical community. It is intertwined with every part of being a physician: dealing with daunting diseases and complex patient cases as an attending physician; learning countless skills in new and uncomfortable situations as a medical student and resident; and navigating a perilous academic road as a premed to even reach medical school in the first place. Life as a physician demands that readiness to step up and face the challenge during tough times. This spirit is emblematic of the road to becoming a physician and life as a physician itself.

But there will inevitably be times when you are knocked down, when your medical career or life itself delivers a blow that makes your knees wobble. It is how you respond in these moments that will shape your path in life. I find that often we remember these experiences most vividly, as they leave the most lasting impression on our hearts and minds.

As I reflect on the decade or so of education and training which led to my current practice as a hospital medicine physician, I can't help but smile while I recall so many poignant memories. There have been countless triumphs as well as tribulations along the way, and both have made the experience unforgettable. In many ways, the most challenging moments of my life have been the most impactful on my development, shaping me into who I am today. Medical training was no exception. Through a mixture of effort and enjoyment, frustration and fulfillment, adversity and achievement, the experience of becoming a physician has been the ride of a lifetime.

Through my reflection, I unearthed some lasting memories, two of which I would like to share with you in this book's final chapter. In doing so, I hope to portray two key snapshots of my experience which are very different from one another. As you will see, I was two very different premeds at these separate inflection points on my journey. Of course, these experiences are not comprehensive; but they do help capture the essence of my journey, the arc of my path within the medical universe. I hope they allow readers to envision my overarching story. I hope they help you better understand at least one example of the varied road to becoming a physician, which is full of ups and downs. Ultimately, bringing that story to light to empower future generations of aspiring physicians is what inspired me to write this book

Chapter 17: A Tale of Two Premeds

I first set foot on the campus of UCLA in 2008 and was immediately enamored with the culture and energy of the place. It had a sort of magic, an excitement which ignited my spirit. I quickly felt that this place was home, and that I would build some of my most lasting memories there. I was not wrong—to this day I can trace many of my best friends, fondest memories, and most valuable lessons back to my time as a UCLA Bruin.

As an incoming freshman, I had chosen biology as a major and intended to pursue medicine as a career. Whether by pure chance, the grace of some higher power, or the values instilled in me by my parents, I fortunately had a strong work ethic that allowed me to perform fairly well academically. I think I knew from the time I was in high school, and certainly during college and beyond, that I was intelligent but certainly never the smartest person in the room. But through hard work and relentless hours perfecting my craft (studies in this instance), I knew that I could perform to the best of *my abilities*. I could rest easy knowing that I had put in the work and done *my very best*, regardless of the actual outcome. That was always my approach to studying: the hard work somehow liberated me from the outcome, or at least made it easier to accept the result knowing I had put forth my best effort. Luckily, this was good enough for both my conscience as well as the standards needed to successfully traverse the perilous premed gauntlet. But the path was not always smooth. One particularly difficult experience is seared in my memory—I will absolutely never forget how I felt that day.

On a Monday morning during the latter part of my very first quarter at UCLA, I suddenly jolted up in bed, covered in a cold sweat. My eyes darted around the room and immediately found the red numbers on my alarm-clock radio (which I used as my alarm back then in the pre-smartphone days). In an instant I felt that lurching sensation in the chest, as if my heart went on break for a moment, leaving my body flailing in limbo. The time read 8:35 AM. My Calculus midterm had started at 8:00 AM sharp.

I couldn't believe my eyes. My mind did not want to admit that this could be happening. *No, no, no, please let that be wrong*, my brain raced in a panic. I ran over to the clock to make sure it was functioning properly and the time was right. I checked my flip-phone and my heart sunk further as the time was indeed 8:35 AM. I simply had not set my alarm correctly. In all my years to that point, this had never happened to me once; but on this fateful day my eyes were not deceiving me. I was about fifteen minutes away from missing the entire duration of an exam which made up a third of my grade. There was simply no other way to state it: I was horrified.

In an absolute blur, faster than I ever had before, I changed clothes, popped in a piece of gum (in all honesty I was so panicked that I didn't even brush my teeth), threw on my shoes, and made a break for it. I absolutely *sprinted* the approximately one-mile route from my dorm room on "The Hill" at UCLA to the lecture hall on the other side of campus. I arrived right around 8:45 AM, as many students were handing in their papers for this fifty-minute exam.

In a frenzy, I sped to the front of the lecture hall, gathered what little composure I had left, and asked the professor if I could have a word. I let him know that I was terribly sorry, and that I took full responsibility, but I had accidentally set my alarm incorrectly and overslept. I asked (as I had never asked for anything before) if I could possibly take the exam late. The professor stood back stoically as I appealed with every morsel of my being, essentially begging for his mercy. The way I remember it, his face revealed not a single shred of emotion. He was a statue. After hearing me out, he said one line and one line only, which I will never forget to this day: "Part of succeeding in my class is being on time." Without another word, he turned on his heel and marched to the other side of the lecture hall. I was stunned. This was nothing short of a roundhouse punch to my soul.

It was clear from his demeanor that there was no reasoning or discussion which could fix this. I understood that the professor was resolute in the decision not to allow me to take the exam. This was clearly evident from the manner in which he delivered this forceful reply. Immediately, my heart dropped to a place it rarely goes. Panic, sadness, worry, guilt—I am not sure what best describes my emotions at that moment, but there were pieces of all of them swirling inside me. I walked outside the lecture hall, attempting to gather myself as best I could. After a moment's pause, my mind and body quickly went back into fight-or-flight mode, searching for a solution to this disaster. I knew the professor had office hours at 9:00 AM immediately after our lecture time. *Surely, I can gather my thoughts, go in there, and ask—or plead—again for a second chance?*

And so I did just that. I had no other choice. I hurried over to the professor's door as soon as his 9:00 AM office hours began, just minutes after my initial heartbreak. Unfortunately, he held as firm as his initial response, which I had fully expected though I wished for a different outcome. I could not repeat the exam, he stated. I would be awarded zero out of one hundred points on this midterm; there simply was no room for excuses in his class. I heard him loud and clear, but somehow my mind was still in disbelief as it grasped for a possible escape from this calamity.

As I walked out of his office around 9:10 AM, reality began to sink in. I had failed an exam in terrific fashion, unlike ever before. There was no doubt that this was the clear low point of my academic career thus far. I sat on the curb in front of a planter and buried my face in my hands. I'm typically not much of a crier, but tears streamed steadily and silently from my eyes in that moment.

My mind raced to some serious thoughts. I already knew the pressure of being a premed at UCLA, of getting the best grades possible from the get-go to avoid falling into an academic hole which would make med school admission impossible. This, of course, was not totally true; medical school admission is much more complex than that and one can overcome great odds on the way to becoming a doctor. But this is how I felt at the time. These were ideas pervading the minds of many premed students, and I was no exception.

I failed, I thought. *A third of my final grade is gone. There's no way I can get higher than a C in this class, and even that would be a miracle if I could pull it off. This is exactly what I was warned not to do: fail early as a premed...What can I do now? What will I tell my parents?*

I'm done for. I won't be able to get into med school because of this.

This last thought, as exaggerated as it was, best encapsulates how I felt in that moment. I was catastrophizing. Clearly the notion was not true; I could still bounce back and succeed going forward. This one mistake would neither define me as a person nor singlehandedly ruin my chance of admission to medical school or any other career path I should choose. But in that moment, this is how I felt, and I felt it strongly. It was terrible, I must admit.

Luckily, though not surprisingly, my parents were extremely supportive. They knew that I was a genuinely dedicated student that had simply made a mistake, one I would have to learn from. They provided me nothing but love and emotional support. I never heard a single reprimand. Though I was hard on myself, this unconditional love was what I needed in that moment. I knew then that parents provide their children something no one else can: unwavering love and support. That is another topic altogether, but it was another powerful feeling that I remember from this time. I felt very fortunate to have them in my corner.

A week went by, dominated by depressive and guilt-ridden feelings, but I tried to bounce back and remain positive as best I could. I did send a follow-up email to my professor. Initially I did not hear back, nor did I expect to; but about a week after the incident, I received a reply. After letting me suffer for several days, apparently to teach me a lesson (as was his right), the professor stated that he would allow me to take a different form of the midterm while he administered an exam for another class.

Praise the lord! I thought. *I have a chance!*

But there was a catch: he would scale my score down by half; in other words, a perfect exam would earn me a maximum of fifty percent.

Ok. Still not the best odds for success...but I'll take it! I thought to myself as I re-read his email reply. *Better than nothing! At least I have a chance to pass this class!*

This solution was tough, but I'll admit that it was fair. I had made a mistake which had consequences, and I had to face those consequences. But I was optimistic. Honestly, at that point, any solution would have been a huge relief and a source of hope, which this certainly was.

If I absolutely crush it from here on out, maybe I can salvage a C or even a B?

The next day (after setting what felt like one hundred alarms), I took the makeup exam and did about as well as I possibly could. I proceeded to bust my tail for the rest of the quarter in that class and every other. I studied hard, as I normally would, but with an added fire in my belly driven by the sheer emotional aftershock of this experience. I wanted to work as hard as I could, leaving no stone unturned when it came to my studies. I wanted to take no chances and control my own destiny. Hard work was the only way I knew to accomplish that, to give myself the best chance of success.

At the end of the quarter, as I opened my student portal to view my grades, I received an incredible surprise. Somehow, some magical way, in the end the professor decided to give me an A in the class. Quite frankly, I was shocked when I saw my grade. I am fairly certain it was a mathematical impossibility for me to achieve that grade with my score on the midterm I had missed, even with the curved test grades we had at UCLA. To this day I do not know for sure, but I think the professor took retrospective pity on me and awarded me this grade because I had worked hard and done as well as I could, given the circumstances.

Ultimately, I will never know. Regardless, I felt so thankful that things worked out the way they did. My gratitude was immeasurable. I had always taken my "profession" very seriously, whether it was school or sports (or later medicine). As an adolescent my passion was always basketball and later in my young adulthood it became my education. Upon enrolling at UCLA, I had decided that I wanted to become a physician. I took that commitment very seriously and I was going to do my absolute best to make it happen. This is why the failure on that midterm hit me so hard. But somehow, good fortune allowed me to emerge relatively unscathed, and in the process, I gained a priceless lesson.

From this experience, I drew a gratitude that further fueled my work ethic. I felt as if there was some divine intervention (I am spiritually oriented but not classically religious) which allowed me to escape failure in this instance. It should not have been possible. It seemed miraculous. But after this experience, I resolved that I would do everything in my power to maximize my potential and do *my very best* in all future pursuits. This good fortune, this free pass if you will, would not go wasted on me. Hard work became my calling card. The universe would be repaid for this karmic gift. Of that, I was sure.

Fast forward to September 2011. I had spent three amazing years at UCLA: living, learning, having a whole lot of fun, and most importantly growing as a person. I had recently applied to medical school and completed my first few interviews. One evening, sitting at my desk in my apartment, I opened my computer and saw an email notification from UCSD School of Medicine. My heart again skipped a beat like it had on the day I missed my midterm; this time it flickered mostly with excitement, but still with a tiny bit of the dread I felt that morning my freshman year. Like any other human being, I hoped for success but also feared failure. This was my med school application decision letter. My first one had finally arrived.

This is it! I thought. *Wow. I can't believe it's here. Could it really happen? But what if it doesn't...*

I pushed this last negative thought from my mind before it could percolate my consciousness. I was going to stay positive. I closed my eyes, took some deep breaths, and said a brief prayer in my head, which always seemed to stabilize me in a highly charged moment.

Ok, here goes nothing. The moment of truth...

I opened the email. I was so excited that my eyes bounced around the page, not reading in a linear fashion. I tended to do that in situations of high tension or excitement. Once I stabilized my eyes and my thoughts, it slowly dawned on me that this was an acceptance letter. I had gotten in! I could hardly believe my eyes.

Yes! YESSSSS! I did it! It all finally paid off! I can't believe it!

I can still remember clearly that I was the only one home in my apartment, as all my roommates were still out and about on campus doing other things. I ran upstairs to the apartment directly above mine where the rest of our closest friends lived (we had the great fortune of all living in the same complex—good times!). I remember barging into their apartment and calling out at the top of my lungs that I got into med school! It was a truly special moment. It was a mixture of joy and relief, both of which are powerful emotions. My friends were elated on my behalf, as they had watched me toil for more than three years in pursuit of this goal. I called my parents and my brother who were overjoyed, as of course they would be. The hard work had finally paid off.

That good fortune I had freshman year—that second chance—was not a waste! I thought to myself. *I did it! Thank you. Thank you.*

I thanked the universe and counted my blessings. It was a special moment for me and my family. I will never forget it.

When I reflect on my time as a premed, these are two of my fondest memories, despite their very different emotional impacts at the time. I recount these two stories in detail partly because they mean something to me, but also to illustrate a point: there was a tremendous arc to my premedical experience, with moments at each end of the emotional spectrum. I went from believing that I was doomed with no chance of med school acceptance to getting into my dream school only three years later. I hope that knowing my experience may comfort you during your own difficult times. We all have a different path to travel, and the journey itself is something to be appreciated. More than an arc, life is really a roller coaster, a sinusoidal wave of ups and downs. But never fret and never fear that failures will prevent you from getting where you want to go. They are not roadblocks but stepping-stones. They will make you stronger.

The pressure on premedical and pre-health students is significant, a fact which I recognize and clearly acknowledge. Some of this pressure is unfounded, as students should have the opportunity to learn and expand their horizons freely without such worries. But inevitably there will be some pressure associated with this educational path, as it is such a competitive field to enter. Getting into medical school and becoming a physician are certainly easier said than done; but, if possible, try to rid yourself of fear of failure or any notion of self-doubt. You *are* capable. You *are* talented. You *can* do it. Through the ups and the downs, stay positive and know that you will make it wherever you want to go (in medicine or otherwise) so long as you keep striving.

Though I was ecstatic upon my acceptance to med school, my journey certainly did not end there. In reality, that was just the beginning of the next chapter in the anthology of a medical career. We are all continually writing our own story books. It is up to us to decide our own destiny, to determine what story will fill those pages. For me, the subsequent chapters of my story included exhilarated learning in med school; intense studying like I had never known when preparing for Step 1 of my boards; the whirlwind of trying to grasp all the medical specialties during my clinical rotations; the thrill of matching at UCSD for internal medicine residency; hours upon hours of hard work as an intern, resulting in immense growth; both stress and satisfaction in my work as a resident; and finally moving on to my current career as an attending hospitalist, which is filled with its own trials and triumphs on a weekly basis. I am still writing my own story, but I am certainly thankful to have ended up where I am today.

In opening this book, I stated that when I started down the road toward becoming a physician, I was somewhat unsure of the best path for my future career. Part of that uncertainty was borne simply from not knowing what a career in medicine would truly hold. I was a perfect example of the premed paradox: navigating uncharted waters with whatever varied bits of information I could gather, resulting in a somewhat incomplete map of my future career. Inevitably there is always some uncertainty as we pursue our goals and progress in life. None of us can be completely sure how any decision will turn out, whether it is what we have for dinner, where we go on vacation, or what we do with our life's work. But what I sought to achieve in writing this book was the following: to help other interested minds attain as much knowledge as possible about the options and experiences that lay before them in the medical field, so that their uncertainty might be a bit more manageable, so that they might find comfort in experience, so that this knowledge might help them along their own journey.

It is my sincere hope that within the pages of this book, we have achieved this goal—together.

References

Chapter 1

1. "2022 Fall Applicant, Matriculant, and Enrollment Data Tables." https://www.aamc.org/media/64176/download?attachment

Chapter 4

1. "Physician Time Spent Using the Electronic Health Record During Outpatient Encounters." https://www.acpjournals.org/doi/10.7326/M18-3684

2. "Tethered to the EHR: Primary Care Physician Workload Assessment Using EHR Event Log Data and Time-Motion Observations." https://pubmed.ncbi.nlm.nih.gov/28893811/

3. "Newton's Laws of Motion." https://www.britannica.com/science/Newtons-laws-of-motion.

Chapter 6

1. "What is Osteopathic Medicine?" https://www.aacom.org/become-a-doctor/about-osteopathic-medicine

2. "US Colleges of Osteopathic Medicine." https://www.aacom.org/become-a-doctor/u-s-colleges-of-osteopathic-medicine
3. "MD vs. DO Programs: Which Path to Medicine is Right for You?" https://elitemedicalprep.com/md-vs-do-programs-which-path-to-medicine-is-right-for-you
4. "MCAT Scores and GPAs for MD-PhD Applicants and Matriculants to U.S. MD-Granting Medical Schools, 2018-2019 through 2022-2023." https://www.aamc.org/media/6151/download
5. "Medical Schools Offering Combined Baccalaureate-MD Programs, by State and Program Length, 2021-2022." https://students-residents.aamc.org/medical-school-admission-requirements/medical-schools-offering-combined-baccalaureate-md-programs-state-and-program-length-2021-2022

Chapter 7

1. "Medical School vs Dental School: How to Choose Your Life Path". https://bemoacademicconsultingcom.lpages.co/medical-school-vs-dental-school/
2. "Dentist Salary in the United States." https://www.salary.com/research/salary/benchmark/dentist-salary.
3. "Pharmacist Salary in the United States." https://www.salary.com/research/salary/benchmark/pharmacist-salary.
4. "Optometry School Cost." https://education.costhelper.com/optometry.html
5. "Occupational Employment and Wages, May 2022: Optometrists." https://www.bls.gov/oes/current/oes291041.htm

6. "What Is the Average Physician Assistant Salary by State." https://www.ziprecruiter.com/Salaries/What-Is-the-Average-Physician-Assistant-Salary-by-State

7. "How Long is Nurse Practitioner School?" https://www.nursingprocess.org/how-long-is-nurse-practitioner-school.html

8. "Where Can Nurse Practitioners Work Without Physician Supervision?" https://online.simmons.edu/blog/nurse-practitioners-scope-of-practice-map/

9. "Nurse Practitioner Salary Guide." https://nurse.org/resources/np-salary-guide/

10. "Nursing Salary By State." https://teach.com/online-ed/healthcare-degrees/online-msn-programs/nursing-salary-by-state/

11. "Physical Therapy Salary and Careers." https://dpt.usc.edu/blog/dpt-physical-therapist-salary/

12. "All About Clinical Psychology." https://www.apa.org/education-career/guide/subfields/clinical/education-training

13. "Occupational Employment and Wage Statistics: Clinical and Counseling Psychologists." https://www.bls.gov/oes/current/oes193033.htm

Chapter 8

1. "Med Schools with the Lowest Acceptance Rates." https://www.usnews.com/education/best-graduate-schools/the-short-list-grad-school/articles/medical-schools-with-the-lowest-acceptance-rates

2. "Table A-1: U.S. MD-Granting Medical School Applications and Matriculants by School, State of Legal

Residence, and Gender, 2022-2023." https://www.aamc.org/media/5976/download?attachment

3. "Premeds: Capitalize on gap years before applying to medical school." https://www.ama-assn.org/medical-students/preparing-medical-school/premeds-capitalize-gap-years-applying-medical-school

4. "Going directly from college to medical school: What it takes." https://www.ama-assn.org/residents-students/preparing-medical-school/going-directly-college-medical-school-what-it-takes#:~:text=American%20Medical%20Association,-Full%20Bio&text=The%20average%20age%20of%20students,so%20directly%20from%20undergraduate%20study.

5. "Age of Applicants to U.S. Medical Schools at Anticipated Matriculation by Sex and Race/Ethnicity, 2014-2015 through 2017-2018." https://www.aamc.org/system/files/d/1/321468-factstablea6.pdf

Chapter 9

1. "Dropping Out of Medical School: Drop Out Rate + Top Reasons." https://financialresidency.com/dropping-out-of-medical-school/#:~:text=According%20to%20the%20Association%20of,between%2015.7%25%20and%2018.4%25.

2. "Step 1: Overview." https://www.usmle.org/step-exams/step-1

3. "Shelf Exams Ultimate Guide (What You Need To Know)." https://themdjourney.com/shelf-exams-ultimate-guide-what-you-need-to-know/

4. "The Socratic Method: Fostering Critical Thinking." https://tilt.colostate.edu/the-socratic-method/

5. "Step 2 CK: Overview." https://www.usmle.org/step-exams/step-2-ck
6. "Top 6 most important factors in getting a residency interview and getting ranked." https://www.medschoolgurus.com/post/top-6-most-important-factors-in-getting-a-residency-interview-and-getting-ranked
7. "4 reasons virtual residency interviews might be here to stay." https://www.ama-assn.org/medical-students/preparing-residency/4-reasons-virtual-residency-interviews-might-be-here-stay
8. "2022 Main Residency Match By the Numbers." https://www.nrmp.org/wp-content/uploads/2022/03/2022-Match-by-the-Numbers-FINAL.pdf
9. "SOAP." https://www.nrmp.org/residency-applicants/soap/.

Chapter 10

1. "ACGME Specialties Requiring a Preliminary Year." https://www.acgme.org/globalassets/pfassets/programresources/pgy1requirements.pdf

Chapter 11

1. "We analyzed 35,000 physician salaries. Here's what we found." https://blog.doximity.com/articles/we-analyzed-35-000-physician-salaries-here-s-what-we-found#:~:text=As%20a%20whole%2C%20academic%20physicians,than%20their%20non%2Dacademic%20counterpoints.
2. "Physician Practice Benchmark Survey." https://www.ama-assn.org/about/research/physician-practice-benchmark-survey

Chapter 12

1. "Is It Better to Be a Doctor Now Than It Was 50 Years Ago?" https://www.mdlinx.com/physiciansense/is-it-better-to-be-a-doctor-now-than-it-was-50-years-ago/
2. "Physician Salaries Declined Over Last Decade." https://journals.lww.com/oncology-times/fulltext/2006/08100/physician_salaries_declined_over_last_decade.9.aspx
3. "Doximity Report: Physician Compensation Growth Not Keeping Pace with Inflation." https://www.healthleadersmedia.com/clinical-care/doximity-report-physician-compensation-growth-not-keeping-pace-inflation
4. "Tuition and Student Fees Reports." https://www.aamc.org/data-reports/reporting-tools/report/tuition-and-student-fees-reports
5. "Average cost of medical school." https://educationdata.org/average-cost-of-medical-school
6. "7 ways to reduce medical school debt." https://www.aamc.org/news-insights/7-ways-reduce-medical-school-debt
7. "AAMC Survey of Resident/Fellow Stipends and Benefits." https://www.aamc.org/data-reports/students-residents/report/aamc-survey-resident/fellow-stipends-and-benefits
8. "How Much Money Do Doctors Make A Year? Doctor Salary By Specialty." https://www.whitecoatinvestor.com/how-much-do-doctors-make/
9. "Physician - Cardiology - Invasive Salary in the United States." https://www.salary.com/research/salary/benchmark/cardiologist-salary

10. "Orthopedic Surgeon Salary in the United States." https://www.salary.com/research/salary/alternate/orthopedic-surgeon-salary

11. "Neurosurgeon Salary in the United States." https://www.salary.com/research/salary/alternate/neurosurgeon-salary

12. "University of California Employee Pay." https://ucannualwage.ucop.edu/wage/

13. "Highest Paid CEOs." https://aflcio.org/paywatch/highest-paid-ceos.

14. "An Introduction to Medical Malpractice in the United States." https://www.ncbi.nlm.nih.gov/pmc/articles/PMC2628513/

15. "Medical Liability Claim Frequency Among U.S. Physicians." 2016. file:///C:/Users/Amit/Downloads/policy-research-perspective-medical-liability-claim-frequency.pdf

Chapter 13

1. "Would You Encourage Your Child to Follow in Your Footsteps and Become a Physician?" https://www.ncbi.nlm.nih.gov/pmc/articles/PMC6143579/

2. "The Future of Healthcare: A National Survey of Physicians." https://www.thedoctors.com/about-the-doctors-company/newsroom/the-future-of-healthcare-survey

3. "Medical Liability Claim Frequency Among U.S. Physicians." file:///C:/Users/Amit/Downloads/policy-research-perspective-medical-liability-claim-frequency.pdf

4. "Medscape Malpractice Report 2017." https://www.medscape.com/slideshow/2017-malpractice-report-6009206#4

Chapter 14

1. "THE HITECH ACT: An Overview." https://journalofethics.ama-assn.org/article/hitech-act-overview/2011-03.
2. "Half of Physician Time Spent on EHRs and Paperwork." https://www.jwatch.org/fw111995/2016/09/06/half-physician-time-spent-ehrs-and-paperwork
3. "Are doctors spending less time with patients?" https://mobius.md/2021/10/09/how-much-time-do-physicians-spend-with-patients/

Chapter 15

1. "Depression: What is burnout?" https://www.ncbi.nlm.nih.gov/books/NBK279286/#:~:text=The%20term%20%E2%80%9Cburnout%E2%80%9D%20was%20coined,ideals%20in%20%E2%80%9Chelping%E2%80%9D%20professions.
2. "Burn-out an 'occupational phenomenon': International Classification of Diseases." https://www.who.int/news/item/28-05-2019-burn-out-an-occupational-phenomenon-international-classification-of-diseases
3. "A crisis in healthcare: a call to action on physician burnout." https://cdn1.sph.harvard.edu/wp-content/uploads/sites/21/2019/01/PhysicianBurnoutReport2018FINAL.pdf
4. "Prevalence of Burnout Among Physicians." https://www.ncbi.nlm.nih.gov/pmc/articles/PMC6233645/

5. "Physician burnout: It's not you, it's your medical specialty." https://www.ama-assn.org/residents-students/specialty-profiles/physician-burnout-it-s-not-you-it-s-your-medical-specialty

6. "A Mindfulness Course Decreases Burnout and Improves Well-Being among Healthcare Providers." https://journals.sagepub.com/doi/abs/10.2190/PM.43.2.b

7. "Mindfulness interventions in medical education: A systematic review of their impact on medical student stress, depression, fatigue and burnout." https://pubmed.ncbi.nlm.nih.gov/29113526/

8. "A systematic review of the impact of mindfulness on the well-being of healthcare professionals." https://pubmed.ncbi.nlm.nih.gov/2875255

About the Author

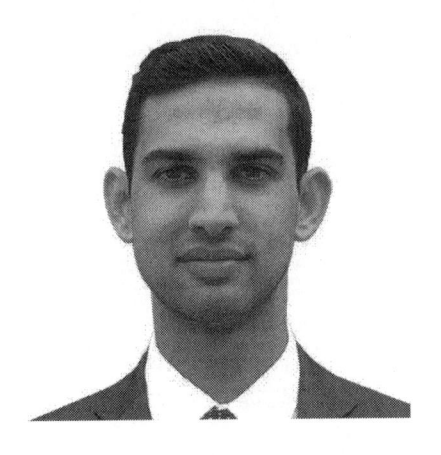

Dr. Amit Pandey is an Internal Medicine Hospitalist with SRS Medical Group in San Diego, California. He attended UCLA for his undergraduate studies followed by UCSD for both medical school and residency. He is Chief of the Division of Hospital Medicine at Sharp Memorial Hospital. Not long ago, he was an excited premed student dreaming about becoming a doctor. Now that he is well into his career, he is passionate about empowering future physicians with the knowledge they need to fully understand a life and career in the medical field. He has extensive experience writing about medical education/training as well as mentoring aspiring premeds. His desire to pay it forward to future generations of physicians, combined with his passion for the written word, inspired him to write this book. Outside of work, he loves to play basketball, exercise, write (of course), and spend time with his loved ones.

Made in the USA
Monee, IL
15 November 2023